The Power
of Stories

The Power of Stories

Nurturing Children's Imagination and Consciousness

HORST KORNBERGER

Floris Books

First published in 2006 by Integral Arts Press, Western Australia
This edition published in 2008 by Floris Books
Second printing 2013

British Library CIP Data available
ISBN 978-086315-659-5
Printed in Poland

Contents

To all those who love stories

Acknowledgments

I would like to thank all my students in story medicine courses and workshops. Without their contributions and enthusiasm the third part of this book would not have been possible. Meg Aldridge, Janet Blagg, Erica Bonsall, Pen Brown, Nandi Chinna, Alejandra Czeschka, Julie Dickinson, John Hamersley, Ute ten Hompel, Jean Hudson, Desma Kearney, Jennifer Kornberger, Leah van Lieshout, Carole Longden, Dianne Marshall, Adrian May, Grace McQuade, Deb Mickle, Tom Muller, Gaye O'Donnell, Kay Rosen, Harriet Sawyer, Aidee Sherrie, Kathleen Shiels, Suzanne Smith, Leanne Sutton, Peter Tenni, Annie Wearne, Mags Webster and Jesse Williamson all contributed pieces of their work.

I would like to express my heartfelt thanks to friend, student and editor Janet Blagg for being the patient midwife to this book and for her forbearance when I substantially revised the manuscript for the third time. Special thanks to Perth storyteller, Jenny Hill, and American storyteller and writer, Nancy Mellon, for important inspiration along the way, to Western Australia craft expert Anne Williams for her beautifully sketched dolls, to Gail Sherback for generously giving her time, Adrian Glamorgan for timely advice and Raymon Ford for his ongoing support. Thanks also to Stefan Szö, who designed the Story Medicine E-book. And last, but not least, to my son Johannes whose hunger for stories inspired this book and my wife Jennifer whose support made it possible.

Author Notes

In this book, stories are taken seriously. I do not aim to present current views about story, rather to show what stories have to say about current views. The result may be surprising to some, but this is the nature of art: to put fuel on burning questions and stir the imagination from its sleep.

Gender switching

I have tried to give equal time to boys and girls, women and men, in my use of the indefinite singular, switching between she and he, his and her, from section to section.

Trading Stories

The Power of Stories is the beginning of a story that has been waiting to be told. For those who wish to become part of this telling I have created a free interactive website for people to share their stories with others.

My desire is to inspire a global artwork arising out of the creativity that each one of us possesses. Its tools are the steps suggested in Part Three of the book and its gallery is the information technology that allows us to communicate with like-minded people all over the world.

If you wish to post your own stories or read stories posted by others, visit our online Community Forums: *http://forums.sofia.net.au*

Introduction

The Ecology of Dragons

Books have their own way of coming into being. This book was born through the meeting of two words: story and medicine.

I have almost forgotten everything about the context in which these words appeared. All I can remember was my feeling of recognition and surprise. I immediately took a pen and made notes. The words opened a floodgate and ideas began to pour out. It was a kind of calling and I immediately followed it. There and then I decided to workshop story medicine.

The two words had met me at the right time. I had lived with stories all my life and witnessed their impact on myself and others. When I was a child stories transported me to another world. As a teenager they allowed me to live a life above and beyond the monotony of everyday events. As an adult they were my trusted friends and mentors — indispensable guides towards who I wanted to become. In hindsight I can see stories standing at every juncture of my life, guiding me.

At the time of meeting the two words I was already teaching creative writing. I have always believed that every human being is creative and I have actively sought ways to further this potential. I had begun to work with a process that allowed my students to experience the essential stages of world literature through their own writing. I soon saw that their creativity was best helped by a minimum of theory and a maximum of story. The more I sifted the great myths and literary works for the life they contained, the more I saw the powerful healing influence that stories have on the lives of those who engage with them.

The words *story medicine* anchored the idea. My first notes became a flyer, the flyer a workshop and the workshop a course. With the help of my students I followed the thread that the words had put into my hand and was led on a journey that became longer and more adventurous as it progressed. My travel journals are contained in this book. What started out as a book about stories and story-making became a book about soul ecology — a manual for inner resource management; action plans to preserve the endangered wildlife of childhood and the biodiversity of the soul in adult life.

There are three parts to this book. The first, 'The Power of Story,' is of general interest, where I set out to think *with* story rather than *about* it. I look at a wide variety of stories and let them speak about their own content. In this way I came across the tale in the tale, a second layer of story encrypted in the first. The tale in the tale is the message in the bottle of story medicine. It is the key that unlocks the secrets of story medicine from antiquity to our time. Using this key, stories reveal themselves as co-creators of cultures, shaping the destiny of whole nations as well as of our individual lives.

The second part of the book, 'Traditional Tales and Their Use,' suggests ways to use the powerful effects of story for the benefit of children and teenagers. It is written for parents, educators, psychologists and all those who want to work with the age-appropriate story as a tool for healing and personal transformation.

Part Three, 'The Making of Stories,' is a manual with detailed instructions for the creation of new stories. It is written for all those who want to develop their skill in story-making. It offers a secure, step by step path towards imaginal capability in a process that mirrors the developmental stages of the imagination itself.

Parts Two and Three comprise a map on which I have charted a temporal landscape of our inner life. The places marked exist in time. The map tells you where to visit with what story and above all, when. For timing is crucial in the practice of story medicine: by telling the right tale at the right time we maximize its healing potential. If we don't place our stories squarely in time, we easily tread the same ground, over and over; slip or even fall.

The importance of the timely story is well illustrated in one of my favourite books, *The Voyage of the Dawn Treader* by C.S. Lewis, in which the author introduces us to a rather nasty little brat, Eustace Clarence Scrubb. Through his education (or lack of it) Eustace Clarence has lived bereft of stories. Whisked away to the imaginary realm of Narnia he is out of his comfort zone and proves utterly useless. Lost on an island he finds shelter in a dragon's lair, but he is not at all prepared:

> Most of us know what we should expect to find in a dragon's
> lair, but as I said before, Eustace had only read the wrong

books. They had a lot to say about imports and exports and
governments and drains, but they were weak on dragons ...

Eustace's inexperience becomes his downfall. In the course of events he
turns into a dragon.

This is not entirely his fault: he has read only the wrong kind of books.
Books that were weak on dragons. And precisely because he had never
heard about them, he became one. The story he did not have had him.

Stories deal with powerful realities. Realities that cannot be dealt with
in other ways. The brittle house of cards of our intellect is of little use
when it comes to dragons. The only way to deal with dragons is to put
them into context. Tales are their natural environment. There they can
safely live and safely die. It is their ecological niche. In it they fulfil a
vital function that cannot be substituted by any other species, imaginative or otherwise. Prematurely extinct, they come to haunt us from
inside. Unaware of them, we do their deeds and don't know why.

Eustace is eventually redeemed. He recovers his humanity from the
dragon nature and returns a better and more caring person. His impact
on the world is changed.

The function of stories is to regulate the household of our soul. They
are part of our interior ecology. They transform, heal and educate the
psyche, and via the psyche the world.

Ecology is the science of interrelatedness. It encompasses the totality of nature as well as the complex environment of the soul. Seen from
this point of view, stories are as much part of the ecological equation as
any other factor of life. A future ecology will no doubt see the parallels
between the spreading of deserts and the desolation of our inner environment. It will recognise them as the same phenomenon and understand
that there is imagination in reality and reality in imagination and that
there is but one great story in which we all partake.

Part 1. The Power of Story

1. The Tale in the Tale

Stories surround us. We can never escape their influence. Our own life is a story in the making and with every deed and decision we continue the telling of it. Our own story is embedded in the larger tale of our time and interwoven with the many tales of all those we meet. We are story-beings and because of it we are often helped by the stories that come our way.

The practice of story medicine is as old as the stories themselves. All ancient traditions used stories as a means of transformation and healing.

American Indian Medicine administered stories alongside herbal remedies. Therapy in classical Greece was embedded in ritual and mythos. The Druids, the healer priests of the Celts, began their training with a long apprenticeship to a bard. In the Sufi tradition tales are used to heal the first and last of wounds — the separation from the divine. The Jewish Sabbath and the Christian mass serve the same purpose: both are stories distilled in ritual and regularly enacted as a means of remembrance and healing.

The steadily growing priesthood of modern psychotherapy also draws on healing tales and myths, and much literature is available on this subject. In this book, however, I avail myself of the theories and explanations from the most authoritative of sources — the stories and myths themselves. For, unrecognised by the reader, many of the great tales contain a complete theory of story medicine written in the fine print of context and between the lines of composition.

The Odyssey

Homer's *Odyssey* provides a classical illustration of story medicine.

> Returning from the sack of Troy, Odysseus is pursued by
> the sea god Poseidon. In vain he tries to reach his home and
> family. For ten years he is tossed on the high seas. He has lost
> all his companions and endured much hardship. Finally, he is
> washed up on the Island of the Phaeacians. The exhausted hero
> is found by the Princess Nausicaa and welcomed at the court
> of her father King Alcinous.

Odysseus gratefully partakes in the hospitality of the Phaeacian king, but does not disclose his identity. During an evening feast, the local bard takes the lyre and entertains the company with a song recalling the quarrel of Odysseus and his compatriot Achilles during the siege of Troy.

Odysseus hears his own tale. He is immediately overcome by emotion and draws his cloak over his head to conceal his weeping. The king notices, but says nothing. On the next evening the bard sings again. This time the theme is the Sack of Troy. Again Odysseus listens to his own story and again he is overcome with emotion. He weeps with such force that the king enquires about his grief.

Once the question is asked, Odysseus reveals himself. He joins again with his destiny and recounts the rest of his story: his ten years of voyage through adversarial seas and the many adventures that lost him his ships and companions. He tells his tale over the remainder of the night. By the approach of dawn, the Phaeacians return the weary Odysseus by means of magical ships back to his beloved Ithaca.

The Odyssey leads us directly into the dynamics of story medicine. Hearing his own story told and then telling the rest of it himself becomes the turning point in Odysseus' life. Homer emphasizes this by placing the encounter of Odysseus with his own story precisely at the culmination of ten years of futile attempts to return home and by following it immediately with his homecoming. All night long Odysseus tells his tale. At dawn he steps into the Phaeacian ship and falls asleep and when he opens his eyes he is back in Ithaca. The return is immediate. The journey is complete.

The composition of the epic reveals the power of story and the importance of timing. Odysseus encounters story medicine when it is its most potent — at the peak of crisis when story can unfold its full potential to transform his life.

The Epic of Parzival

Once the basic pattern or dynamic of story medicine is recognised it can be easily found in other works, for instance the medieval epic of *Parzival*.

Parzival is brought up by his mother Queen Herzeloyde in great seclusion. She wishes to keep him from the dangerous pursuit of knighthood. But as soon as Parzival chances upon two knights, he cannot be constrained. Longing to become a knight he leaves his mother. Through his prowess in battle he soon wins the hand of a princess, lands and high renown. Seemingly at the peak of his career, he is received among the knights of King Arthur's table.

But amid the ensuing celebration, the sorceress Cundrie appears and accuses Parzival of being devoid of honour and a disgrace to the round table. She shames him publicly and curses him for his lack of compassion for the ailing King Anfortas.

She is referring to a time when Parzival had been received hospitably in the castle of the wounded King Anfortas. Parzival had observed the king's agony, but in keeping with the conventional manners he'd been taught, rather than following the promptings of his heart, he had failed to ask the compassionate question, 'What ails thee?' According to a prophecy, that question would have ended the suffering of the king and brought great honour on Parzival.

Now at the height of his success Parzival's failure comes to haunt him. Parzival leaves King Arthur's court in distress. He longs to find the ailing king again and ask the redeeming question, but he searches in vain. He journeys for many years devoid of companionship and the comforts of home and family.

Feeling unfairly treated by destiny Parzival loses his trust in God. Eventually he meets the hermit Trevrizent and takes lodging with him. Their conversation turns toward the Grail and the pious man, ignorant of Parzival's identity, tells his guest the history of the Grail. He ends with the woeful tale of its latest keeper, King Anfortas, and of the opportunity lost by an ignorant youth to redeem his suffering through the question: 'What ails thee?'

Hearing his own story in this way, Parzival begins to understand it in the context of the greater tale — the history of the Holy Grail and the tragic destiny of its keeper Anfortas. He finally realizes the impact of his own failure to ask the compassionate question. His conscience awakens. Owning his story he leaves the hermit and soon finds the Grail Castle and the suffering king. This time he asks the redeeming question and in turn becomes the new Grail King. He unites with his family and the knights of the round table.

There are many striking similarities between the epic of *Parzival* and *The Odyssey*. Both heroes encounter dramatic changes of fortune immediately after reaching the height of success — the fall of Troy, the honour of being admitted at the Round Table. Both journey alone on a long and seemingly unattainable quest. Both find help in the height of their crisis. Both have their story told to them by somebody who is ignorant of their true identity. Both subsequently reveal themselves and tell the rest of their tale and the fortunes of both immediately improve after the encounter with story medicine.

Variations of the pattern can also be detected in the epic of *Gilgamesh*, who has to repeat his life story three times before he reaches the abode of the immortal Utnapishtim. Oedipus, perhaps the most tragic of all heroes, wrestles with his own story as others wrestle with monsters or formidable foes. In the myth of Orestes the hero rids himself of the Furies only by embracing his story and admitting his guilt.

The latest version of liberation through story may be found in the work of the South African Truth and Reconciliation Committee dealing with the atrocities committed during the Apartheid regime. Perpetrators are offered total amnesty for a complete and public disclosure of truth.

Telling the story of their personal part in the greater tale of suppression and racism and hearing it told from the victims' perspective becomes their doorway to freedom. Perhaps the oldest form of story medicine is the Aboriginal songlines, the great creation stories that have shaped the Australian continent. When they are sung, the land hears its own story. Listening to its own genesis the land is restored to its original shape. As different as these stories are in other respects, in their story medicine they are remarkably similar. A pattern is clearly discernible. An archetypal sequence reveals itself. What is the meaning of this pattern? Why does the tale in the tale occur in so many myths? Let us again consult the stories. They themselves will tell us how they want to be understood.

Stories do not explain in a direct way; they show by example. The tale in the tale is this example. Through it, stories reveal their way of working. The tale in the tale is the explanatory manual in which stories show us how they work on the hero. And in showing us how they affect the hero, they are also showing how they affect us, because they affect us in the same way that they affected Odysseus or Parzival — as an agent of change and a catalyst that completes the hero quest. That is, if it is the right story at the right time — for then it pertains to us, is our story and part of our life. This type of story acts like a tale in the tale of our life and helps us to take the next step. The encounter with such a story can take many forms.

It may begin with a new book beckoning enticingly from a showcase. Opening it at home we might find it disappointing and so bury it in the lowest strata of our library. But years later when we find ourselves in crisis and confusion the book catches our eye again and we resurrect it from its dusty grave. We open it and this time we are hooked. Each line seems written just for us. The story it tells speaks to us. It contains the map that disentangles the mess of our life. Stumbling blocks soon look like stepping stones into the new. We move on and are changed.

In the first encounter the story failed to have an impact on us. The message it contained did not pertain to any situation in our life. The content left us cold and unengaged. The medicine it contained was not needed at the time. All this has changed by the second encounter and the story has become a tale in the tale of our life. It affects us in the same way that hearing his own story affected Odysseus. The story has become a catalyst that helps us to take the next step. It is story medicine.

Sometimes the relationship between the content of a story and our life may be blatantly obvious. At other times it may remain unconscious. The intellect may not be able to see the link, but the soul recognises the healing properties of the story like the body recognises a lacking vitamin.

In either case the story will work its way to the soul and unfold its healing potential.

2. Meeting with Story

So far the tale in the tale has shown us how stories can work on us. But it has more to tell. Let us follow it further into the lives of such extraordinary human beings as the Buddha and the Christ.

The religious masters are the ultimate heroes in whose destiny reality and myth, history and story coincide. Archetypal patterns that merely announce themselves in the destiny of mythical heroes are clearly revealed in their lives.

Gautama Buddha

The Buddha was born the son of an Indian king and queen. Buddha is the title that he acquired after his illumination. He was initially named Siddhartha Gautama.

> Siddhartha's birth is accompanied by many auspicious signs and a prophecy that he would become either a great saint or a world ruler. His worldly father prefers the latter and does everything to prevent the spiritual pursuits of his son. The young prince is brought up confined in the luxury of the royal palace to keep him away from the sufferings of the world. Eventually he is married to the princess Yasodhara to tie him to a householder's life; she soon falls pregnant and his father's aim seems fully achieved.
>
> But the gods send four signs. In the palace gardens, Siddhartha chances upon first an aged man, then a sick man and finally a corpse. He awakens to the transitory nature of life and is left with great questions tormenting his soul. Then he glimpses a wandering ascetic and immediately sees what path he ought to follow.
>
> He takes leave of his family and home and becomes a wandering monk, travelling the lands with shaved head, robe and begging bowl. He apprentices himself to various spiritual teachers, but soon masters all they can teach. Disappointed and

disillusioned with the limitations of what he has learned, he
embarks on a regime of harsh austerity, living on one sesame
seed and one grain of rice a day. But severe asceticism does
not grant him the enlightenment he longs for and after six
years he renounces all extremes and returns to the life of a
wandering monk.

Finally Siddhartha sits down under the sacred Bodhi tree
and vows not to rise again until he has achieved enlightenment.
He remains there for forty days and sinks into ever deeper
states of meditation.

But before attaining enlightenment, he is confronted by
Mara, the infernal god of this world, and his three sensual
daughters, attempting to seduce him from his goal. When
this fails, Mara attacks him with an army of demonic monsters and beasts. The earth convulses and violent winds break
loose. The demons unleash all the evil powers at their command, hurling huge rocks and hot coals, axes and spears,
sand and mud, but nothing touches the calm of his concen-
trated mind.

Mara leaves defeated and Buddha enters a deep state of
meditation. In the clarity of his undisturbed mind, he sees all
his many lives spread out before him and realizes his own
place in the history of Bodhisattvas. Then he penetrates the
laws of karma and the four 'noble truths' that will be the
cornerstone of his doctrine, and finally the boundless, death-
less realm of liberation; Nirvana, the final goal. He does not,
however, remain there, but out of compassion returns to the
world to share his insight.

After the years of failure and the terrifying assaults of Mara, the Buddha
is confronted with his whole story. His story contains more than one life,
and he surveys the sum totality of his many incarnations to the last and
final breakthrough in one grand vision, which he immediately follows
by attaining his ultimate goal of total enlightenment. This is the perhaps
the highest expression of story medicine, the realization of the highest of
goals: total liberation and the outpouring of compassion. It is Buddha's
compassion alone that keeps him from fully leaving this earth.

Jesus Christ

If we look into the life of Christ we again find story medicine in the height of crisis, when Christ, nailed to the cross, utters:

> Eli, Eli, lamashabach tany.
> 'My God, my God, why hast thou forsaken me?'

This is no cry of despair. It is the first line of Psalm 22, a psalm so famous at the time that this line was enough to evoke the whole psalm and all the meanings and hopes associated with the coming of the Messiah. It is one of the psalms of King David, poet and prophet, written 800 years before Christ invoked it on the cross.

> My God, my God, why hast thou forsaken me? Why art thou so far from helping me, and from the words of my roaring? O my God, I cry in the daytime, but thou hearest not; and in the night season, and am not silent …
>
> But I am a worm, and no man; a reproach of men, and despised of the people.
>
> All they that see me laugh me to scorn: they shoot out the lip, they shake the head, saying, He trusted on the Lord that he would deliver him: let him deliver him, seeing he delighted in him …
>
> Be not far from me; for trouble is near; for there is none to help.
>
> Many bulls have compassed me: strong bulls of Bashan have beset me round.
>
> They gaped upon me with their mouths, as a ravening and a roaring lion.
>
> I am poured out like water, and all my bones are out of joint: my heart is like wax; it is melted in the midst of my bowels.
>
> My strength is dried up like a potsherd; and my tongue cleaveth to my jaws; and thou hast brought me into the dust of death.
>
> For dogs have compassed me: the assembly of the wicked have inclosed me: they pierced my hands and my feet.
>
> I may tell all my bones: they look and stare upon me.

> They part my garments among them, and cast lots upon my
> vesture.
> But be not thou far from me, O Lord: O my strength, haste
> thee to help me ...

Psalm 22, Authorized Version

The description of suffering bears little resemblance to David's life. His hands and feet were never pierced. Nobody ever parted his garments or cast lots upon his vestures. It is prophetic.

In quoting this psalm Christ consciously fulfils the story he has come to tell and he tells it in the moment of fulfilment. Hearing and telling coincide in a fully conscious act that completes the gospel of self-knowledge that heroes like Oedipus and Odysseus began. Like them, Christ turns for home immediately after telling his story: he exchanges his temporal existence for eternal life.

The Buddha fulfilled his mission as a Bodhisattva and the Christ fulfilled the Hebrew prophesies of the Messiah that lace the scriptures from the first book of Genesis to the last book of the prophets.

The unreserved and fully conscious meeting with one's own story is obviously the mark of the great spiritual masters that have graced the earth. The meeting with one's own story is a heroic act that takes courage and maturity. Without these, the story may be heard, but not recognised. Or it may be recognised, but rejected.

The rejection of story and the implications of such rejection have been carefully investigated by one of the great psychologists of the modern era, William Shakespeare.

Hamlet

The young Prince Hamlet administers a good dose of story medicine to his usurping uncle, King Claudius, who he suspects of having murdered his own father to obtain the crown and queen. Hamlet seeks final proof, and to obtain it he stages a play before Claudius, a play depicting the murder he suspects his uncle to have committed.

The effect of the play is immediate. The king pales and storms away. Hamlet has his proof, the king his story. We soon find Claudius in the chapel, praying.

> O, my offence is rank, it smells to heaven;
> It hath the primal eldest curse upon it;
> A brother's murder!

The play has made Claudius acutely aware of his crime, but still he clings to his ambition, to the fruits of his deed.

> Pray I cannot, though inclination be as sharp as will ...
> What form of prayer can serve my turn? Forgive me my 'foul
>   murder'?
> That cannot be; since I am still possess'd
> Of those effects for which I did the murder,
> My crown, mine own ambition, and my queen.

It is brilliant self-analysis, but coupled with an incapacity to change. And so the tragedy marches on towards its bitter end. The story that could not change Claudius, however, changes the play. It becomes the turning point for the tragedy and the catalyst for everything that follows.

For Hamlet's sole aim is to avenge his father, not to make his uncle repent. To achieve repentance, a different kind of story medicine is needed.

David and Bathsheba

The use of story medicine to bring about repentance is illustrated in the biblical tale of King David and Bathsheba. The physician is no less than the Hebrew God himself.

King David, standing on the roof of his house, sees the beautiful Bathsheba in a neighbouring garden. She is the wife of Uriah, one of the king's officers. David falls in love with her and, while her husband is away at war, has Bathsheba brought to him. When she falls pregnant David tells the commander of his troops to put Uriah into the front line. When Uriah is killed in battle David takes Bathsheba as one of his own wives.

This displeased his god.

> And the Lord sent Nathan unto David. And he came unto him,
> and said unto him:

'There were two men in one city; the one rich, and the other
poor. The rich man had exceeding many flocks and herds: But
the poor man had nothing, save one little ewe lamb, which he
had bought and nourished up: and it grew up together with
him, and with his children; it did eat of his own meat, and
drank of his own cup, and lay in his bosom, and was unto him
as a daughter. And there came a traveller unto the rich man,
and he spared to take of his own flock and of his own herd, to
dress for the wayfaring man that was come unto him; but took
the poor man's lamb, and dressed it for the man that was come
to him.'

And David's anger was greatly kindled against the man; and
he said to Nathan: 'As the Lord liveth, the man that hath done
this thing shall surely die: And he shall restore the lamb fourfold, because he did this thing, and because he had no pity.'

And Nathan said to David: 'Thou art the man. Thus saith
the Lord God of Israel, I anointed thee king over Israel, and
I delivered thee out of the hand of Saul; And I gave thee thy
master's house, and thy master's wives into thy bosom, and
gave thee the house of Israel and of Judah; and if that had been
too little, I would moreover have given unto thee such and
such things. Wherefore hast thou despised the commandment
of the Lord, to do evil in his sight? Thou hast killed Uriah the
Hittite with the sword, and hast taken his wife to be thy wife,
and hast slain him with the sword of the children of Ammon.'

II Samuel 12:1-9

The device is similar to that in Shakespeare's play, but the Hebrew God
is more subtle than Hamlet. Yahweh's aim is repentance and healing and
it is to this end that he uses the parable. When David hears the story, he
does not realize that it pertains to him. He is outraged to hear of such
injustice. In his righteous anger he demands death for the perpetrator.
Only then does the prophet Nathan disclose the truth. David is shattered. He repents deeply. Being the darling of his god and a great poet
of penitent psalms saves his life, though calamity later catches up with
him when his own son Absalom deals with him as treacherously as he
dealt with Uriah.

Nathan's administration of story medicine allowed David to feel enraged
about his own injustice. The tale made space for righteous anger to arise.

The story Nathan tells is one of the first parables in world literature. The parable is a major means of story medicine. Like all effective remedies it is tailored to a situation at hand, and unlike direct accusation, it does not address the problem explicitly. Parables forego accusation and do not preach; they use imaginative means instead, evoking metaphors of a situation, pictures of a moral dilemma.

Through the use of story the parable separates the perpetrator from the deed. Unknowingly, the king listens to what he has done and so becomes a witness to his own acts. This allows his higher self to sit in judgement over his lower affairs.

Parables always call on independent judgement. They are a statement of trust in the inviolable morality of the essential human being. They have the effect of real remedies rather than symptomatic cures; they activate the innermost source of health and let it take effect.

In the case of King David the parable became the story medicine that helped him to take a step that King Claudius could not make.

The Prodigal Son

The Old Testament contains only few parables, but the gospels are full of them. The founder of the Christian faith is one of the most productive story-makers of all time. He pioneers the parable as a major healing tool.

The parables of Christ are immediate story medicine, situational and remedial; they are poetic improvization on the roadside, at the dinner table, the inn; unpremeditated and straight from the heart.

Christ's use of parable is no accident; the parable is complementary to his mission. According to the Christian faith, Christ is a divine being descended into human reality. He is a god that walks in the common garb of humanity. The parable does the same: it embodies divine truth in simple pictorial form. A true disciple of its master, the parable speaks the vernacular of the soul, a language that everybody can understand. It touches the heart and bypasses the complications of religious laws. Like the story of Nathan it calls on the higher self but does not force it into obedience. It leaves men and women free to respond from their own core.

Jesus uses parable and poetic metaphor like a master physician uses remedies. He makes tinctures of poetic medicine in the language of the soul — illuminating, healing and challenging. His parable of the prodigal son is a masterpiece in the medicinal use of story. He tells this tale to the Pharisees and Scribes, the religious and intellectual establishment, who turned against him because he mixed with publicans and sinners. He uses the parable to challenge their opposition.

> Likewise, I say unto you, there is joy in the presence of the angels of God over one sinner that repenteth.
>
> And he said, A certain man had two sons: And the younger of them said to his father, Father, give me the portion of goods that falleth to me. And he divided unto them his living. And not many days after the younger son gathered all together, and took his journey into a far country, and there wasted his substance with riotous living.
>
> And when he had spent all, there arose a mighty famine in that land; and he began to be in want. And he went and joined himself to a citizen of that country; and he sent him into his fields to feed swine. And he would fain have filled his belly with the husks that the swine did eat: and no man gave unto him. And when he came to himself, he said, How many hired servants of my father's have bread enough and to spare, and I perish with hunger!
>
> I will arise and go to my father, and will say unto him, Father, I have sinned against heaven, and before thee, and am no more worthy to be called thy son: make me as one of thy hired servants. And he arose, and came to his father. But when he was yet a great way off, his father saw him, and had compassion, and ran, and fell on his neck, and kissed him. And the son said unto him, Father, I have sinned against heaven, and in thy sight, and am no more worthy to be called thy son. But the father said to his servants, Bring forth the best robe, and put it on him; and put a ring on his hand, and shoes on his feet. And bring hither the fatted calf, and kill it; and let us eat, and be merry: For this my son was dead, and is alive again; he was lost, and is found. And they began to be merry.
>
> Now his elder son was in the field: and as he came and drew nigh to the house, he heard music and dancing. And he called one of the servants, and asked what these things meant. And he said unto him, Thy brother is come; and thy father hath killed

the fatted calf, because he hath received him safe and sound.
And he was angry, and would not go in: therefore came his father out, and entreated him. And he answering said to his father,
Lo, these many years do I serve thee, neither transgressed I at
any time thy commandment: and yet thou never gavest me a kid,
that I might make merry with my friends: But as soon as this thy
son was come, which hath devoured thy living with harlots, thou
hast killed for him the fatted calf. And he said unto him, Son,
thou art ever with me, and all that I have is thine. It was meet
that we should make merry, and be glad: for this thy brother was
dead, and is alive again; and was lost, and is found.

Luke 15:10-32

The parable of the prodigal son goes further than mere illustration. It is
a complete story, a miniature drama with all the ingredients of a therapeutic artwork whose intention is the ultimate healing or homecoming
of the human soul. Its core is the transformation of the hero through a
process in time. The parable is too short to contain another tale — the
tale in this tale is shrunk to the squanderer's realization of his miserable
state and his repentant return.

With its archetypal strengths and parabolic completeness, I see the
parable of the prodigal son as the structural ancestor of later fairytales.
Like them it contains many layers of meaning — at its highest level, no
less than the destiny of humanity from the beginning of the world to its
end; the journey from Paradise to the heavenly Jerusalem.

Those with a fine ear to the ancestry of story will hear the prodigal
son returning in *Hansel and Gretel*, in *Cinderella* and in *Little Red
Riding Hood*. He comes home in every tale that ends with the hopeful
'And they lived happily ever after.'

Tongues of Fire

Christ's ability to speak in parables seems to have had its own dynamic
of death and resurrection. It appears to perish with him, then resurfaces
at the Whitsun event, when his disciples are seized by the Holy Spirit.

And when the day of Pentecost was fully come, they were
all with one accord in one place. And suddenly there came a

sound from heaven as of a rushing mighty wind, and it filled
all the house where they were sitting

And there appeared unto them cloven tongues like as of
fire, and it sat upon each of them. And they were all filled with
the Holy Ghost, and began to speak with other tongues, as the
Spirit gave them utterance.

And there were dwelling at Jerusalem Jews, devout men,
out of every nation under heaven. Now when this was noised
abroad, the multitude came together, and were confounded, because that every man heard them speak in his own language.

And they were all amazed and marvelled, saying one to
another, Behold, are not all these which speak Galileans? And
how hear we every man in our own tongue, wherein we were
born?

Suddenly the disciples can speak a language everyone understands.
This gift of tongues lives powerfully among the early Christians and then
disappears again, drowned in the dogma of the organized church.

If we look for the resurrection of this gift in later times we find it in
the great stories of humanity. For *when these stories are noised abroad,
the multitude comes together, and is confounded, because every man and
woman hears them speak in their own tongue.*

The great tales speak a universal tongue that transcends boundaries of
nations, religions and languages. This is nowhere more obvious than in
the world-wide and lasting appeal of fairytales. If anything has preserved
the gift of tongues, it is the fairytale, understood by everyone in their
own way. Fairytales speak in the global tongue of pictures and in the
language of homecoming that has its origins in the parables of Christ.

3. The Mother of Myth

We have begun our journey with the tale in the tale, the story medicine that allowed the homecoming of the heroes and the completion of their quest. We recognised this tale as a manual through which stories reveal themselves and their way of working. We met with the essence of story medicine in the lives of Buddha and Christ. There the tale in the tale unfolded its full potential as a catalyst of destiny and a last rung on the ladder of spiritual ascent. We also looked at the rejection of story and how it may be remedied through the parable.

So far we have seen the influence of story on individual lives. The tale in the tale, however, has more to tell. Rightly read it reveals the greater mission of myth and its impact on a people. For each myth is a tale in a greater tale. It belongs to a whole body of myths. There it fulfils the same function as the tale in the tale fulfils in *The Odyssey* — it becomes a means of transformation and change.

In this way *The Odyssey* not only affects the life of an individual, but that of a whole people. It is story medicine for the culture it belongs to. It is a tale in the tale of Greek myth. It is part of a large body of myth in which all stories are intertwined.

Nowadays, we come to know these stories one by one. We don't live in them as they once were lived in: we meet them in isolation. It is as if we had found a finger or nose of a broken sculpture. But if we come to know a sufficient number of myths we may become more aware of the intricate mythological universe of which they are part.

A body of myth is like a complete poem cycle, a grand artwork, an epic tale. Every single myth is a tale in the tale of this large body of stories. The myths that feature most prominently often present a culture with pictures of its destiny long before this destiny becomes reality. They prepare the remedy long before the illness comes about. Cultures take millennia to mature. The great myths are the mothers who bring them to birth and give of themselves to prevent cultural stagnation.

The great stories, therefore, stand at the inception of cultures such as India, Egypt and Greece, and not at their end. They are the co-creators, mothers, guides and instructors of what is to come. Myths prepare the ground for what is achieved later. They are cause rather than effect, seeds sown in the fertile soil of the human psyche, already containing the germ that will shape itself in the course of time.

Imagination precedes reality like a mother her child. This is particularly clear if we look at the Greek myths that foreshadowed all the major contributions of classical Greece. They were pregnant with the brainchild of philosophy long before its birth in historic time. It was Greek myth that induced the change from the old, magical and matrilineal mode to that of conscious thought. What Greek philosophers achieved in the time between Thales and Aristotle was prepared in the stories of Theseus and the Minotaur, Perseus and Medusa, and the Battle with the Centaurs.

Theseus and the Minotaur

The story of Theseus and the Minotaur tells how the young Theseus, son of King Aegeus of Athens, liberates his city from a cruel tribute.

> Every year seven boys and girls are shipped to Crete and there devoured by the Minotaur, a bull-headed monster lurking in the depths of a labyrinth.
>
> Theseus resolves to challenge the monster and offers himself as substitute for one of the boys. When he arrives in Crete, Ariadne, the daughter of King Minos, falls in love with him. To aid the young hero, she bestows a sacred gift on him: a spool of thread to lead him in and out of the labyrinth.
>
> Theseus winds out the thread to the centre of the labyrinth. There he confronts the bull-headed monster and kills him in combat. Then, by means of his thread, he retraces his way back through the dark maze, to the light of day. The Minotaur is dead and the spell broken. The tribute is now forfeit and Athens is liberated from the domination of Crete.

> Crete is the perfect location for this myth. On this long stretch of island that lies between the aged wisdom of Egypt and the bold beginnings of Greece, an ancient, magical and matrilineal culture preserved itself in exceptional purity and strength.
>
> The Minoans retained a wisdom beyond conscious grasp, a highly developed culture from pre-individualistic times: har-

monious though not free, wise though not conscious, powerful
but a power achieved without effort. Even now we can feel
the echoes of paradise rippling through their playful designs,
their innocent portrayal of women and men; we can marvel at
their total lack of fortifications, the absence of any evidence of
conflict, and the enviable balance between the sexes.

In Minoan Crete the bare-breasted queen holds the snakes of
initiation, and young men and women somersault effortlessly
over the sacred bull.

At first sight this portrayal of a gracious Crete may seem at odds with a
myth depicting a dangerous labyrinth and a bull-headed monster feeding on innocent youth. The paradox makes sense when we realize that
the myth represents the Athenian fear of the hypnotic power of the past,
manifest in the confusion of the labyrinth. The bull-headed Minotaur
stands for the pre-conscious, instinctual wisdom that would devour the
new impulses emerging in Greece.

Not unlike the new generation who rebel against everything their
parents hold dear, the Greeks secured their mission through the rejection of the culture that came before theirs. This process is reflected in
the way Theseus overcomes the labyrinthine wisdom of Crete: he does
so with the help of a thread — that is, through the fine-spun linearity of
thought. (Even nowadays we speak of the thread of thought and of the
confusion that reigns when it is lost.) To complete his quest, Theseus
kills the Minotaur — the inspired, instinctual, bull-headed forces that
would overpower the emergence of a new mode of thought centred in
the head.

I can only marvel at the precision of this myth, its prophetic direction
and initiatory power that reaches right down into the spirit of place. The
tale situates the emergence of thought in Athens, long before Socrates,
Plato and Aristotle made it the undisputed centre of philosophy. With the
subsequent development of philosophical logic and science, the unravelling of the Greek thread was complete.

Athens itself derives its name from Pallas Athene, the Greek goddess
of wisdom who emerged fully formed from the cleaved head of her
father Zeus. It is not surprising that the goddess who emerged idea-like
from her father's head is the patron of philosophers and the protector of
the city that housed the famous schools of philosophy.

Perseus and Medusa

The myth of Perseus and Medusa tells the same tale from a different angle.

> Perseus is charged with the task of beheading the snake-haired Medusa. This is an almost impossible feat, as everyone who looks at her is immediately turned to stone.
>
> But he is helped by Pallas Athene with good advice and helpful tools, among them a polished shield with which he approaches the sleeping Medusa, walking backwards. Viewing her indirectly in the reflection of his shield, he is guarded from the impact of her gaze.
>
> Using his shield as a mirror, he severs her head and hides it in a sack. At this point Pegasus, the winged horse, emerges from the monster's body and takes to the air.

The Medusa is like the Minotaur. In each of them the head — the centre of thought — is obscured by the instinctual forces that governed the past. The snakes wriggling on Medusa's head represent the vital life animating the unconscious soul, the power of old initiations, the complicated wisdom of the pre-individuated mind. The Medusa wears her labyrinth on her head. She is an ancient creature; her power is enormous, hypnotic and real. Whoever gazes on her is turned to stone; lost in the bewildering maze of her animistic wisdom, further movement towards self-conscious thought is halted.

Perseus cunningly uses his shield as a mirror. This approach is well considered: he overcomes the sleeping Medusa by means of reflection — itself a perfect picture for the use of thought. For thought mirrors reality and so dulls its impact. Thinking always kills the life of immediate experience.

What Perseus first achieved has long since become our second nature. We follow his approach whenever we reflect on reality until we are clear of the wriggling snakes of confusion.

In this story we are again confronted with the transformation of the old into the new, from imaginal consciousness into rational thought. But there is a surplus in the power of the Medusa: a mighty, vital, primeval force that resists neat constructs of thought; something that cannot be contained in the straitjacket of categories or the linearity of philosophy's proofs. This power is Pegasus, the winged horse of fantasy, imagination and art. In Pegasus the power of Medusa is resurrected into new life.

And while Medusa's tumultuous snakes are gone, their vitality still animates the swelling columns of every temple, the subtle life of sculpture and the pulse of Greek poetry.

The Battle with the Centaur

The centaurs are among the earliest inhabitants of the Greek imagination, half-human, half-beast. From the waist upwards they share the human form, while the lower part of their body is that of a horse. Through this constitution they partake deeply in the knowledge and instinctual wisdom of the past, a quality that makes them master physicians. Generally they are benevolent and caring. When they are drunk however, they lose conscious control over their instinctual nature. Then their unbridled urges run wild and they try to violate the bride, the virgin soul, the new forces emerging in classical Greece.

> The centaurs are invited to the marriage feast of King Pirithous and his bride Hippodamia. During the feast the half-human creatures get intoxicated with wine. Losing control they try to rape the women. The king and his guests, among them Theseus, take arms. In the ensuing battle the Greeks are aided by Apollo, the god of balance, harmony, music and conscious restraint. Inspired by his presence the heroes overcome the centaurs and rescue the women unharmed.

The whole of Greek culture is one long battle with the centaur — a slow emancipation from the past through the process of overcoming what is instinctual by means of the thoughtful control of the self.

The Centaur in The Odyssey

Often we find the imagination of the centaur hovering almost imperceptibly over the most sublime creations of classical antiquity.

Homer's work, which links prehistoric myth with historic reality, is a grand exposition on the theme of the centaur. He treated this theme in the manner of true story medicine: it is written entirely in the invisible ink of composition. The battle with the centaur is encoded in the contrast between *The Iliad* and *The Odyssey*, Achilles and Odysseus.

The two epics are as distinct as their two heroes. In spite of its length, the Iliad describes only a short incident in the ten year siege of Troy. Its subject matter is the fierce anger Achilles holds for Agamemnon, the leader of the expedition, and the consequences of Achilles' withdrawal from battle. *The Odyssey*, by contrast, spans the ten years of Odysseus' attempts to return to Ithaca after the fall of Troy. Achilles is the last of the mythical heroes; Odysseus the forerunner of a new age.

Achilles is the son of the goddess Thetis and possesses the supernatural strength of a demi-god, except for the spot at his heel left vulnerable by his mother at birth. He is brought up by the centaur Chiron who rears the young hero on a diet of lion, boar and bear. He is the unmatched champion of the Greeks in their war against Troy.

Through his origin and upbringing Achilles is tied to the mythical past. The forces of the centaur are alive in him. He is easily overpowered by his emotions. The epic centres on his wrath, the elemental power of his anger that almost ruins the whole expedition. Only when Patroclos falls in battle does he rejoin the action, his fury over the loss of his beloved companion overcoming his anger with Agamemnon. Drunk with rage he hurls himself back into battle, wreaking carnage among the defenders of Troy.

Odysseus is of very different character. His origin is purely human and he boasts no supernatural strength. He excels in the very qualities that Achilles lacks: caution, foresight, cunning and self-control. He is a man of ideas, a warrior with the sword of thought.

After ten years of battle it is not Achilles' supernatural strength that wins the war, but Odysseus' cunning idea to hide within the Trojan horse. He accomplishes in days what ten years of warfare failed to achieve.

In his adventures on his way home after the fall of Troy, it is his capacity to use his head that continually saves him from harm. He escapes the one-eyed giant Polyphemus through his inventiveness. He saves his ship through his cautious approach to the land of the Lastrygones. He is clever enough to escape the snares of the sorceress Circe and wise enough to follow her advice when appropriate. He shows foresight by tying himself to the mast of his ship before approaching the enticing song of the Sirens. He knows how to keep his vessel to the safe middle path between the sea monsters Scylla and Charybdis. When his companions slaughter the sacred cattle of Helios, he shows his power of restraint by foregoing the meal and so saves himself from the stormy revenge of the god. Even when the nymph Calypso tempts him with the prospect of immortality, he does not lose sight of his goal to return home.

Put *The Iliad* and *Odyssey* side by side and the centaur emerges in epic form. In Achilles the semi-divine horse-like powers of the past hold sway. In Odysseus the conscious forces rise above the instincts, much like the human part of the centaur rises above his rump. Odysseus is a philosopher in action, a thinker in deeds. Take all his virtues, add philosophical thought to them, and the *Ethics* of Aristotle is almost complete.

When, thousands of years after the first inception of this myth, Socrates withstands the seduction of Alcibiades, the most handsome, brilliant and desirable young man in the whole of Athens (homosexuality was favoured among educated Greeks), the myth is fulfilled and the centaur overcome. Philosophic composure has won the battle against instinctual urge.

And when, some years later, the unjustly condemned Socrates refuses to violate Athenian law in order to save his life, the last hairy hoof of the centaur morphs into an elegant toe.

4. The Magnitude of Loss

In the last chapter we encountered the directive power of myth. We saw how in three different stories the destiny of ancient Greece announced itself in myth long before it became reality. The stories, however, tell only one side of this tale. They celebrated the victory of conscious thought without elaborating on the price that was paid for it. Greek myths have equally much to say about the pain incurred in the process. The stories of Cassandra, Medea and Orestes describe the magnitude of loss, but no myth explores the painful dimension of this loss more acutely than the story of Oedipus.

Oedipus and the Price of Self-knowledge

Laius and Jocasta, the royal couple of Thebes, have been child-less for many years. King Laius asks the oracle of Delphi for advice and is forewarned by Apollo not to have a son, for that son would kill his father and marry his mother.

Alarmed, the king resolves to shun the bed of his wife. Feeling abandoned, Jocasta reverts to cunning: at a feast she makes Laius drunk and once more they share a bed. When nine months later Oedipus is born, Laius tears the baby away from its mother, pierces his feet with a sharp nail, and orders a shepherd to abandon the wailing child in the mountain wilderness.

The crying babe, however, is found by a shepherd from the neighbouring kingdom of Corinth. Moved by pity he takes the wounded child and presents him to the childless king and queen of Corinth. They adopt the baby as their son and name him Oedipus, wounded foot.

Oedipus grows up a prince of Corinth and heir to the throne.

When the young prince is taunted by some drunken peers that he bears little resemblance to his parents, he begins to be plagued by doubt. To resolve the riddle of his origin he makes a pilgrimage to Delphi. But when he poses his question, the priestess reproaches him, calling him cursed, for he will murder his father and marry his mother.

Oedipus is shattered. In order to avoid the fulfilment of the oracle he resolves never to return to Corinth. He turns towards Thebes instead.

While he is making his way from Delphi to Thebes, Laius is coming from Thebes to Delphi, also to seek advice from the oracle. A sphinx, a creature that is half-woman, half-winged lioness, plagues the city. She waylays travellers and poses them a riddle that no one can solve, then devours her helpless prey.

The two travellers meet on a tight mountain pass. The king, sitting in his royal chariot, calls out to the wanderer to make way for his betters. The young prince replies that he acknowledges no betters than the gods and his own parents.

Laius orders his charioteer to drive straight on and not mind the youth, and the wheels of the chariot roll over Oedipus' feet. Angered and pained by his wounded feet, Oedipus spears the charioteer, pulls Laius from his seat, entangles him in the reigns of his own horses and whips them until they drag the king to his death.

Oedipus continues on his way to Thebes and is waylaid by the sphinx, who poses her riddle: 'What is it that walks on four legs in the morning, on two legs at noon and on three legs in the evening?'

When Oedipus answers: 'The human being,' the riddle is solved. The defeated sphinx hurls herself from a cliff. The city is liberated and Oedipus is welcomed as a hero. When the news of King Laius' death arrives, Oedipus is offered the crown and marries the widowed queen Jocasta. The oracle has been fulfilled.

Ignorant of the noose that is tied around his neck Oedipus becomes King of Thebes and proves a just and capable ruler. Two sons and two daughters are born from his union with Jocasta: Eteocles and Polyneices, Antigone and Ismene.

After some years a plague afflicts the city of Thebes. Oedipus sends messengers to the oracle of Delphi for advice and the oracle announces that the pestilence is caused by the unrevenged murder of King Laius. Oedipus, who has remained ignorant about his part in the deed, proclaims a life-long punishment for the perpetrator and dedicates himself to the search for the murderer.

The evidence mounts to reveal his own abysmal entanglement, the deadly sin committed through his ignorance, the incestuous union with his mother and the misshapen fathering of his own siblings. Maddened by despair Jocasta hangs herself and Oedipus, seized by the agony of his shame, pierces out his eyes.

Oedipus takes on the sentence of banishment and leaves Thebes to lead the life of a blind and homeless beggar, assisted by his daughter Antigone. When the aged Oedipus requests permission to return to Thebes, his sons refuse him. Finally, the suffering hero finds refuge with Theseus, King of Athens.

The oracle that once declared him cursed now announces that he is blessed, and that when he dies his remains will make supreme the country in which they are buried. Now his ambitious sons try to force his return to Thebes, but Oedipus withstands their attempts and remains in Athens under Theseus' protection.

As a hero, Oedipus is closely related to Theseus, Perseus and Pirithous. He too faces a half-human creature, the sphinx, who he overcomes by means of his intellect. Only the intellect, which can distinguish human beings from the beasts, is able to give answers and solve riddles. The myth hints at this through the very response that destroys the sphinx: the human being.

The life of Oedipus is one long and painful meeting with the pitfalls of the intellect, the shortcomings of human reasoning. The myth of Oedipus is the myth of the intellect and therefore of ignorance; of the total blindness that goes hand in hand with the power of thought. From the beginning of the myth to the end we are confronted with the helplessness of human endeavour, the shortcomings of reason, the utter inadequacy of the intellect when faced with the powers of destiny. Oedipus is the first martyr of the mind, and a monument to the futility of reasoning.

Being the myth of the intellect, Oedipus is also, inevitably, the creation myth of irony. No other myth is as painfully and consistently ironic. Irony is conceived in the gap between our understanding of a situation and the actual fact of that situation, a gap that the intellect with its limitations necessarily creates.

Thus Laius does all within reason to avoid the conception of a child and in consequence brings about the very thing he tried to prevent. What a marvellous proof of ignorance.

When the newborn Oedipus is pierced through his feet and left to perish in the wilderness, the theme repeats itself with a new layer of tragedy and pain — and this is only the overture to the great drama that is to unfold when Oedipus himself is confronted with the prophecy. Now it is the hero who, by trying to avoid his destiny, runs straight into it. We see him caught in a breathtaking acceleration of events, stumbling helplessly within the vicious dance of his fate.

He turns towards Thebes and immediately meets the father he sought to avoid. The myth emphasizes their mutual ignorance in the bitter irony of their exchange:

'Make way for your betters.'

'I know no betters than the gods and my parents.'

The knot tied by destiny finally becomes a noose when Laius' chariot crushes Oedipus' feet, the very feet that Laius had pierced with a nail. It is as if the feet remember the pain the head had forgotten. In his rage Oedipus fulfils the prophecy he so desperately tried to escape.

Through the language of composition the myth reveals the price that must be paid for the acquiring of intellect: the death of the father and incestuous marriage with the mother. It is no coincidence that the murder of his father immediately precedes and the incest with his mother immediately follows Oedipus' conquest of the Sphinx.

His intellectual victory is flanked by two devastating losses. Both stand for the loss of the older, imaginal cognition, the instinctual knowing that would have recognised mother and father even if they had never been met.

But the myth has not yet reached its culmination. The final cruel exposure of human ignorance arises through a masterstroke of destiny when Oedipus is made to search for the murderer of King Laius.

Now he becomes the first detective: an investigator against himself. What greater evidence of ignorance can there be than to be searching for oneself and not know it. And what greater irony than to pursue a murderer and find it is oneself.

By means of his clever intellect Oedipus painfully discovers how ignorant his intellect really is. In one devastating moment of self-knowledge the truth is revealed. Oedipus pierces his eyes to acknowledge his blindness. His intellect thought it could defeat the powers of destiny but ends up prostrate at destiny's feet. It seems fitting that Theseus of Athens, who reaped the benefits of intellect's emergence, should shelter the martyr who suffers its painful consequences.

And so the myth returns us to Athens, to the city that will keep the remains of Oedipus after his death and so also retain the blessings of his life. For it is in Athens that the prophecy attached to Oedipus is fulfilled, by one of the great philosophers of antiquity, one in whom intellect was exalted and redeemed: Socrates.

Socrates and The Dialectics of Irony

The destinies of the mythical hero and the historical philosopher complement each other, first of all through the oracle of Delphi that played a powerful part in the shaping of both their lives.

In the pronouncement that Oedipus will kill his father and marry his mother, the oracle marks him as the most ignorant of men. By contrast, Socrates is pronounced the wisest of all the Greeks.

The oracle of Delphi catapults Oedipus into the thicket of his destiny, and urges Socrates on in his philosophical quest. But what marks Socrates as the heir of Oedipus' blessing is revealed in his philosophical method.

The oracle made Oedipus investigate his own delusions and so discover how ignorant he really was. Urged by the same oracle, Socrates does the same to his philosophic adversaries. Engaging their intellect he pushes them to discover how deluded their intellect is. Like Oedipus they end up confronted with their own ignorance.

In the Socratic dialogues the drama of Oedipus repeats itself in the arena of philosophic thought. Here it is both fulfilled and redeemed. Even the irony that so bitterly ruled Oedipus' life becomes servant to the mind of the great philosopher. Socrates' *Apology* is a masterpiece of ironic rhetoric delivered before the court of Athens, where Socrates stands accused on false charges. In its opening lines we can see that the myth has become integrated.

> What effect my accusers have had upon you, gentlemen, I do
> not know, but for my own part I was almost carried away by

them; their arguments were so convincing. On the other hand, scarcely a word of what they said was true. I was especially astonished at one of their many misrepresentations: the point where they told you that you must be careful not to let me deceive you, implying that I am a skilful speaker. I thought that it was peculiarly brazen of them to have the nerve to tell you this, only just before events must prove them wrong, when it becomes obvious that I have not the slightest skill as a speaker — unless, of course, by a skilful speaker they mean one who speaks the truth. If that is what they mean, I would agree that I am an orator, and quite out of their class.

The tragedy of Oedipus becomes the tragicomedy of Socrates. Through Socrates, western civilization reaped the benefits of Oedipus' suffering. While all later philosophy rests upon the contributions of Socrates, Plato and Aristotle, their work rested squarely on the directive power of Greek myth. To lack awareness of what we owe to the mythical past is to repeat the sin of ignorance and bring down the curse of Oedipus, not his blessing.

Whether or not they are tragic, myths play their role in the shaping of culture. With a close reading, their impact is precise and tangible. The stories of Oedipus, Theseus and Odysseus helped transform the rough heroes of the Trojan War into the thoughtful philosophers of later times.

On a greater scale a complete mythology like the Greek or Norse does the same for the whole of humanity: it serves as a tale in the tale within the great global story, a catalyst for the next step that humanity has to take. This makes all stories our stories and every culture a source of the story medicine we all need. Indian myths open up like lotuses on the calm lake of ancient spirituality. The Persians weighed good and evil on the scales of their tales. The Babylonians saw through the telescope of story back to the creation of the stars. The Egyptians made their myth step into the coffins of stone and the Greeks began to thread thought into the labyrinth of their tales. Each myth has its own voice in the choir of global tales.

5. The Twilight of the Gods

The Shaping of Myths

The link between myths and reality, ancestral story and historic achievement remained unconscious in the early Greeks. The old faded as the new gradually emerged. Only in hindsight do the connections become apparent. The same holds true for most cultures and their myths. The great tales are the overture to the drama that every culture performs on the world stage. Creation myths are particularly telling in this respect.

> Indian creation myth begins with Vishnu lying motionless on the thousand-headed cobra which floats on the ocean of milk. His first deed is to emanate his sakti, his divine counterpart and wife, Lakshmi, the goddess of abundance and harmony. From Vishnu's navel a pink lotus flower emerges on a long stalk. In the lotus Brahma is seated. The newborn Brahma searches for the reason of his own existence, and that of the universe. Vishnu appears to him and advises him to undergo fervent austerities. Brahma takes the advice and in intense meditation he creates the inner heat from which all other gods and demons arise. Once the gods are created they commence with the creation of the world.

This is only the beginning of the myth, but already it contains the central themes of Indian culture — the master–pupil relationship, spiritual practice and severe austerity. Brahma himself sets the precedent for the unending line of spiritual masters and gurus that kept that aspect of India alive over millennia. While other ancient cultures faded away the spiritual life of India continued to thrive.

Ancient Egypt, for instance, has entirely sunk into the tombs it made for itself. It is not surprising to find the theme of entombment is a major motif in Egyptian myth.

The Egyptians trace themselves to Ra, the self-created god, who with the power of his words created the world. When he had spoken everything into being, Ra descended unto the earth and ruled Egypt for many thousands of years. But eventually he began to grow old and his bones became like silver, his flesh like gold and his hair like lapis lazuli. Bent by age he could no longer fight Apophis, the dragon of evil lurking in the vapours of night. And so he passed his rule to his children Isis and Osiris. But Osiris's evil brother Set is envious of his throne and plots his death.

Set has a chest made of precious wood to fit the proportions of Osiris. He then invites his unsuspecting brother to a splendid feast and promises the precious chest to whatever god may fill its size. Osiris lies down and finds the chest a perfect fit. In this moment Set slams the door, nails it down and seals all cracks with lead. The chest becomes his coffin. Set throws the chest into the Nile and the waters carry it far away to the city of Byblos. After a long search Isis finds the body of her husband and brings it back to Egypt.

But evil Set learned her secret. Coming in the night, he snatched the body of Osiris and tore it in fourteen pieces, scattering the parts all over Egypt. Eventually Isis finds the scattered parts and buries each on in a different part of the land.

The themes of age and death, coffins and tombs, dominate these myths. Ra turns into metal and stone and Osiris dies in a coffin. Torn into pieces he is buried in fourteen different tombs. Egypt had a rare passion for death and almost all the artifacts that have been excavated from its numerous tombs were made to be viewed by the dead and not by the living. The whole culture followed its gods into the grave.

Even the sober Romans could not escape the shaping myth. They lacked true myth and so became uniquely unimaginative and artistically unproductive. Thus myths fulfil themselves, even through their absence.

The Lost Myth

But what of our own myths? Where are they and how have they shaped our lives? Are we as ignorant about their influence as the Greeks were about the directive power of their tales? To answer these questions we must occupy ourselves for a while with Norse mythology — the grim ancestor of our fairytales and of the original stories of western culture. (Norse myths were by no means restricted to Scandinavia. They were common to most tribes that migrated across Europe.)

Nordic myth, or Germanic myth, is the forgotten myth of Western culture. It is powerful fare, painted in the fierce contrast between light and dark, peopled with gods, giants, dwarves, elves, witches, Valkyries and warriors; a myth in which the conflict between giants and gods spans all time, from the beginning of the world to its cataclysmic end known as the Ragnarok, the Twilight of the Gods.

This twilight is foreshadowed by the death of the beautiful Baldur, the most beloved of all gods.

> Baldur is the son of the god-father Odin and the goddess Frigg. When Odin has a foreboding dream about his son's death, Baldur's mother exacts an oath from all beings never to harm her son. She asks everyone except the harmless mistletoe growing high in the branches of trees. Once all beings have given their word, the gods play a game of jest by hurling their weapons at the invulnerable Baldur. But the envious and scheming Loki, the treacherous friend of the gods, carved an arrow from the mistletoe. He then made Baldur's blind brother Hodur partake in the jest and shoot the arrow at Baldur. The beautiful god is struck and dies.
>
> With Baldur gone all goodness and piety flees from the world and the gods know that they are doomed.
>
> The Norse myths end with the god-father Odin listening to the prophecies of the Vala, the seeress of the Germanic tribes. The Vala foresees the twilight of the gods that cannot be avoided now that Baldur is dead.
>
> In this Twilight even the gods are destroyed. The giants gather and storm Valhalla, the heavenly stronghold of the gods. Evil is unleashed. God-father Odin faces the Fenriswolf and is mauled in its jaws. His son Thor suffocates in the poisonous fumes of the Midgard snake, the hissing serpent of evil. Hodur battles with the treacherous Loki until both are killed. The gods fall, the earth shakes, storms are unleashed, tidal waves devour the land and fire bursts loose. The light *is* drowned in darkness. Only few survive, among them Vidar, the silent Aesir

who avenges his father Odin on the Fenriswolf and who will
raise a new world from the ashes of the old. Then Baldur, so it
is said, will return again from the realm of the dead and make
his abode among the living.

Norse myths are tragic. The Twilight of the Gods is the blood pulsing
through the body of Germanic tales. It is the dark mark made at the
birth of time, the curse brought down at the beginning of creation when
the gods killed the giant Ymir and made mountains and rocks from his
bones, fashioned the sea from his blood and the sky from his skull. This
was the deed that sowed enmity between the gods and the giants and
sealed the fate of the world.

From this moment on the gods live with the knowledge of their
impending destruction at the end of time. Even they cannot escape, only
bide their time and prepare for the final battle, Ragnarok. They live,
feast, adventure and fight in the shadow of doom, their destiny woven by
the Norns, the great mothers at the root of the world tree, Yggdrasill.

Today, Vili and We, Baldur and Hodur, Bragi and Iduna have all
disappeared. For many in the English-speaking world their existence is
at best marginal. Norse myth has fulfilled its own prophecy and extinguished itself from the consciousness of those who once owned it. The
myth has died the heroic death of its own making.

By contrast, Aphrodite and Ares, or, in their Roman incarnations,
Venus and Mars, have lost little of their appeal. Oedipus is a complex.
Eros is omnipresent and Psyche has merged with soul. And the familiar
presence of the Greek gods and heroes is matched by those of biblical
tradition: Adam and Eve, Cain and Abel, Moses and Miriam, David and
Bathsheba, Solomon and the Queen of Sheba, the life of Christ and Mary
and the apostles, martyrs and saints.

The Nordic apples of Iduna could not compete with the apple grown in
the fertile soil of Paradise. Relatively few know anything much of Thor,
though Samson is still going strong. Except for occasional appearances in
Wagner's operas, the Norse gods have disappeared from the stage.

The Loss of the Imagination

But myth does not die so easily. The stories may go underground, the
names get lost, the pictures dissolve and contents fade, but the life of

myth goes on. It returns under the mask of ordinariness and reclaims new territory for the spectres of the past. We met the vengeful return of story in the Introduction, where Eustace Clarence Scrubb became a dragon because the story he did not have had him. The effect of such unconscious stories is not restricted to individuals.

Myths act in the same way on the soul-life of a people, a culture or an age. The life of myths spans millennia. Their biography is history. Their crises are wars, their achievement is culture. Their expression is the reality we know. Myths cannot be avoided. Ignored, they are most often fulfilled by those who heed them least.

This is nowhere more obvious than in Nordic, or Germanic, myth.

Outwardly it has waned. But its end is only apparent, for its waning is part of its own grand design. When the Twilight of the Gods was only a prophecy, it was the vision of the Vala, a foreseeing of doom.

Now the prophecy is fulfilled. The Norse gods are gone and their vibrant world has vanished. Their myths have disappeared according to their own prophecy. Our present culture is the living expression of Ragnarok. In our way of seeing the world we have extinguished the gods and their stories. Thus Germanic myth has only apparently ended: it culminates in our time and in our experience of the world.

In this world Baldur is dead. Our imagination is gone. The intellect has taken its place. This is the Twilight of the Gods. Our seemingly rational culture is the current expression of its mythical plan. Even our rational reduction of myth to mere fancy is an element of the Twilight of the Gods. We live in the middle of a myth we know nothing about.

The loss of this myth is part of a greater story, the story made by the Mother of Myth. Myth is her story behind history; history is the intellect's reading of it.

6. The Return of the Imagination

The loss of story, of the lived reality of myth and of imagination, is the culmination and fulfilment of Norse myth, but not all the gods died in its cataclysmic end. Vidar and Vale survived, and together with Baldur who returned from the dead, they create a new and better world.

If we look for a new kind of story rising from the ashes of the old tales we find it in the European household or fairytales. These tales are to the Nordic stories what Vidar and Baldur are among the gods — a new and happier generation. Though their forebears were doomed, they live 'happily ever after.' The household tales redeem their Nordic ancestors. They do not deny the death of Baldur or the Twilight of the Gods that follows in its wake, but they do not end there.

In the tale of *Sleeping Beauty* the death spell of the thirteenth fairy is transformed into a hundred-year sleep. And though the sleep cannot be avoided, Beauty and the rest of the court will awake at the appointed time.

Like Odin, Little Red Riding Hood falls prey to the wolf. But unlike the Nordic god she is not mauled in his jaws. The hunter will retrieve her alive. Snow White appears to be dead and is laid out in a coffin of glass, but she too is revived in the end. Norse myth emphasizes death, the fairytale resurrection.

The famous collection of the Brothers Grimm contains over two hundred stories. Among the most popular are those that address the twin themes of death and resurrection — the death of Baldur and his return after the Twilight of the Gods.

Donald Mackenzie in *Teutonic Myth and Legends* describes Baldur thus:

> Baldur the Beautiful was the most noble and pious of all the gods in Asgard. The whitest flower on earth is called Baldur's brow, because the countenance of the god was snow-white and shining. Like fine gold was his hair, and his eyes were radiant and blue. He was well loved by all the gods, save evil Loki, who cunningly devised his death.

The parallels between Baldur and heroines like Snow White and the Sleeping Beauty, who are beautiful, pious and well-loved by everyone except their stepmother or the evil fairy, are obvious. Baldur's brow is as white as the heroine of the famous fairytale. His mother who exacts an oath from all beings not to harm her son is like the father of the Sleeping Beauty who orders all spindles in his realm to be burned in order to keep her from harm. But just like the Ragnarok, the hundred years of sleep cannot be avoided.

Many of the famous heroines of fairytales suffer Baldur's fate — the fate that the imagination invariably suffers in the Twilight of the Gods: the extinction of its own world and of the stories within it.

We are living in the middle of this extinction. We partake in the old and the new. The world-wide popularity of tales like *Sleeping Beauty* and *Snow White* supports this observation. They are popular because they mirror our predicament. Fairytales are the story medicine of Western culture. We unconsciously recognise ourselves in the heroines of these tales. We suffer what they suffer and hopefully succeed where they have succeeded before us — in the resurrection from death of the imagination.

To do this we must follow their lead to a deeper understanding of the twilight of the imagination in our soul. We must come to understand the effect of Ragnarok in ourselves and in our culture. We can do this with the help of a story that directly deals with the loss of story that comes with the Twilight of the Gods. The Goose Girl is one of the tales collected by the Brothers Grimm in the first half of the nineteenth century.

The Goose Girl

There was once upon a time an old queen whose husband had been dead for many years, and she had a beautiful daughter. When the princess grew up she was betrothed to a prince who lived at a great distance. When the time came for her to be married, she had to journey forth into the distant kingdom, and the aged queen packed up her many costly vessels of silver and gold, and trinkets also of gold and silver, and cups and jewels, in short, everything which appertained to a royal dowry, for she loved her child with all her heart.

She likewise sent her maid-in-waiting, who was to ride with the princess and hand her over to the bridegroom, and each had a horse for the journey. The horse of the king's daughter was called Falada, and could speak.

So when the hour of parting had come, the aged mother went into her bedroom, took a small knife and cut her finger with it until it bled. Then she held a white handkerchief to it into which she let three drops of blood fall, gave it to her daughter and said, dear child, preserve this carefully, it will be of service to you on your way.

So they took a sorrowful leave of each other, the princess put the piece of cloth in her bosom, mounted her horse, and then went away to her bridegroom. After she had ridden for a while she felt a burning thirst, and said to her waiting-maid, dismount, and take my cup which you have brought with you for me, and get me some water from the stream, for I should like to drink. If you are thirsty, said the waiting-maid, get off your horse yourself, and lie down and drink out of the water; I don't choose to be your servant.

So in her great thirst the princess alighted, bent down over the water in the stream and drank, and was not allowed to drink out of the golden cup. Then she said, ah, heaven, and the three drops of blood answered, if this your mother knew, her heart would break in two. But the king's daughter was humble, said nothing, and mounted her horse again.

She rode some miles further, but the day was warm, the sun scorched her, and she was thirsty once more, and when they came to a stream of water, she again cried to her waiting-maid, dismount, and give me some water in my golden cup, for she had long forgotten the girl's ill words. But the waiting-maid said still more haughtily, if you wish to drink, get it yourself, I don't choose to be your maid. Then in her great thirst the king's daughter alighted, bent over the flowing stream, wept and said, ah, heaven, and the drops of blood again replied, if this your mother knew, her heart would break in two.

And as she was thus drinking and leaning right over the stream, the handkerchief with the three drops of blood fell out of her bosom, and floated away with the water without her observing it, so great was her trouble. The waiting-maid, however, had seen it, and she rejoiced to think that she had now power over the bride, for on losing the drops of blood, the princess had become weak and powerless.

So now when she wanted to mount her horse again, the one

that was called Falada, the waiting-maid said, Falada is more suitable for me, and my nag will do for you, and the princess had to be content with that. Then the waiting-maid, with many hard words, bade the princess exchange her royal apparel for her own shabby clothes, and at length she was compelled to swear by the clear sky above her, that she would not say one word of this to anyone at the royal court, and if she had not taken this oath she would have been killed on the spot. But Falada saw all this, and observed it well.

The waiting-maid now mounted Falada, and the true bride the bad horse, and thus they travelled onwards, until at length they entered the royal palace. There were great rejoicings over her arrival, and the prince sprang forward to meet his bride, lifting the waiting-maid from her horse, thinking she was his consort.

The waiting-maid was conducted upstairs, but the real princess was left below. Then the old king looked out of the window and saw her standing in the courtyard, and noticed how dainty and delicate and beautiful she was, and instantly went to the royal apartment, and asked the bride about the girl she had with her who was standing down below in the courtyard, and who she was. I picked her up on my way for a companion, give the girl something to work at, that she may not stand idle.

But the old king had no work for her, and knew of none, so he said, I have a little boy who tends the geese, she may help him. The boy was called Conrad, and the true bride had to help him tend the geese. Soon afterwards the false bride said to the young king, dearest husband, I beg you to do me a favour. He answered, I will do so most willingly. Then send for the knacker, and have the head of the horse on which I rode here cut off, for it vexed me on the way. In reality, she was afraid that the horse might tell how she had behaved to the king's daughter.

When she succeeded in making the king promise that it should be done, and the faithful Falada was to die, this came to the ears of the real princess, and she secretly promised to pay the knacker a piece of gold if he would perform a small service for her. There was a great, dark-looking gateway in the town, through which morning and evening she had to pass with the geese: would he be so good as to nail up Falada's head on it, so that she might see him again. The knacker's man promised to do that, and cut off the head, and nailed it fast beneath the dark gateway.

Early in the morning, when she and Conrad drove out their flock beneath this gateway, she said in passing, alas, Falada, hanging there.

Then the head answered, alas, young queen, how ill you fare. If this your mother knew, her heart would break in two.

Then they went still further out of the town, and drove their geese into the country. And when they had come to the meadow, she sat down and unbound her hair which was like pure gold, and Conrad saw it and delighted in its brightness, and wanted to pluck out a few hairs. Then she said, blow, blow, thou gentle wind, I say, blow Conrad's little hat away, and make him chase it here and there, until I have braided all my hair, and bound it up again.

And there came such a violent wind that it blew Conrad's hat far away across country, and he was forced to run after it. When he came back she had finished combing her hair and was putting it up again, and he could not get any of it. Then Conrad was angry, and would not speak to her, and thus they watched the geese until the evening, and then they went home. Next day when they were driving the geese out through the dark gateway, the maiden said, alas, Falada, hanging there.

Falada answered, alas, young queen, how ill you fare. If this your mother knew, her heart would break in two.

And she sat down again in the field and began to comb out her hair, and Conrad ran and tried to clutch it, so she said in haste, blow, blow, thou gentle wind, I say, blow Conrad's little hat away, and make him chase it here and there, until I have braided all my hair, and bound it up again.

Then the wind blew, and blew his little hat off his head and far away, and Conrad was forced to run after it, and when he came back, her hair had been put up a long time, and he could get none of it, and so they looked after their geese till evening came.

But in the evening after they had got home, Conrad went to the old king, and said, I won't tend the geese with that girl any longer. Why not, inquired the aged king. Oh, because she vexes me the whole day long. Then the aged king commanded him to relate what it was that she did to him. And Conrad said, in the morning when we pass beneath the dark gateway with the flock, there is a horse's head on the wall, and she says to it, alas, Falada, hanging there.

And the head replies, alas, young queen how ill you fare. If this your mother knew, her heart would break in two.

And Conrad went on to relate what happened on the goose pasture, and how when there he had to chase his hat.

The aged king commanded him to drive his flock out again next day, and as soon as morning came, he placed himself behind the dark gateway, and heard how the maiden spoke to the head of Falada, and then he too went into the country, and hid himself in the thicket in the meadow. There he soon saw with his own eyes the Goose Girl and the goose-boy bringing their flock, and how after a while she sat down and unplaited her hair, which shone with radiance. And soon she said, blow, blow, thou gentle wind, I say, blow Conrad's little hat away, and make him chase it here and there, until I have braided all my hair, and bound it up again.

Then came a blast of wind and carried off Conrad's hat, so that he had to run far away, while the maiden quietly went on combing and plaiting her hair, all of which the king observed. Then, quite unseen, he went away, and when the Goose Girl came home in the evening, he called her aside, and asked why she did all these things. I may not tell that, she said, and I dare not lament my sorrows to any human being, for I have sworn not to do so by the heaven which is above me, if I had not done that, I should have lost my life.

He urged her and left her no peace, but he could draw nothing from her. Then said he, if you will not tell me anything, tell your sorrows to the iron stove there, and he went away. Then she crept into the iron stove, and began to weep and lament, and emptied her whole heart, and said, here am I deserted by the whole world, and yet I am a king's daughter, and a false waiting-maid has by force brought me to such a pass that I have been compelled to put off my royal apparel, and she has taken my place with my bridegroom, and I have to perform menial service as a Goose Girl: if this my mother knew, her heart would break in two.

The aged king, however, was standing outside by the pipe
of the stove, and was listening to what she said, and heard it.
Then he came back again, and bade her come out of the stove.
And royal garments were placed on her, and it was marvellous
how beautiful she was. The aged king summoned his son, and
revealed to him that he had got the false bride who was only a
waiting-maid, but that the true one was standing there, as the
former Goose Girl. The young king rejoiced with all his heart
when he saw her beauty and youth, and a great feast was made
ready to which all the people and all good friends were invited.

At the head of the table sat the bridegroom with the king's
daughter at one side of him, and the waiting-maid on the other,
but the waiting-maid was blinded, and did not recognise the
princess in her dazzling array. When they had eaten and drunk,
and were merry, the aged king asked the waiting-maid, as a
riddle, what punishment a person deserved who had behaved
in such and such a way to her master, and at the same time
related the whole story, and asked what sentence such a person
merited. Then the false bride said, she deserves no better fate
than to be stripped entirely naked, and put in a barrel which is
studded inside with pointed nails, and two white horses should
be harnessed to it, which will drag her along through one street
after another, till she is dead.

It is you, said the aged king, and you have pronounced your
own sentence, and thus shall it be done unto you. And when
the sentence had been carried out, the young king married his
true bride, and both of them reigned over their kingdom in
peace and happiness.

The Homeopathy of Story

Folktales are potent remedies. They are the homeopathy of story medicine: small in size but vast in impact. Accurate mirrors of inner dynamics, like homeopathy they treat like with like.

Bearing multiple meanings, they may also be likened to a holographic
image which, due to the nature of light, contains the whole picture within
any one of its parts. If the whole is broken, even the tiniest part preserves

the original image, even if with less clarity. So, due to its inner light, the folktale preserves its meaning, even in partial interpretations.

Even at the most elemental level of interpretation, the tale of the Goose Girl can be applied to almost any problem without losing its integrity. For most of our problems have, like the Goose Girl, lost their story. They are entities in isolation and they behave like imposters. As problems, they present themselves as the true reality and take our place in assuming the role of self. When we put them in context they are solved; they regain their story, their true place in the bigger picture.

The Tale as Parable of the Soul

At the next level of interpretation The Goose Girl can be seen as a parable of the soul. From this perspective, all the characters of the story reveal themselves as aspects of our inner life, and the composition of the tale becomes transparent for the stages of our inner development.

The queen mother stands for the best part of our past, for all that is familiar, supportive and safe — our mother, family, home, childhood. Leaving home we take our gifts, which are always magical (the handkerchief, the talking horse). The princess represents the best part of our self and the maid the worst.

The journey is life itself. It takes us away from home and into strange and unfamiliar places where we are stopped by the false maid, the skilled usurper of our intentions. It is she who takes away our story and with it our true identity, for our story is who we are. We are forced to deny ourselves until we find our true story again — the one that puts everything into perspective and that exposes the imposter.

The Goose Girl contains a tale in the tale. In it the heroine finds her own story and through her own story, her self.

But what does it mean to find one's own story? How do we access story medicine? In answering this, the layer of interpretation pertaining to our own life links with the next layer of meaning in the tale. Like all great stories The Goose Girl is not just a personal tale, but one of humanity.

Our story is never our story alone. It is always linked with other tales. It is most likely part of a greater tale we know little or nothing about. The story of the Goose Girl is linked to the tales of her mother and her maid, and to the stories of the king and of Conrad and her bridegroom.

Her story is part of a greater tale that unites her with all who touch upon her destiny. By contrast, the false tale imposed on her by the maid keeps her in constant isolation.

Consider also the myth of *Parzival*. The story that helps him on his quest is not his story alone. The tale that Trevrizent tells the young knight begins in heaven with the fall of Lucifer and leads by way of Adam and Eve to the grail kings and the tragic Anfortas, and ends with Parzival's missed opportunity to redeem the ailing king. The hermit unfolds a spiritual history from the beginning of the world to the point of their meeting. Only against the backdrop of this greater tale does Parzival's own story become meaningful and healing. It is the greater tale that brings him home.

When Buddha sees all his many incarnations spread out in front of him he realizes his place in the long line of Bodhisattvas. He sees his own story as part of the greater tale of Eastern spirituality and so finally becomes the Buddha, a fully illumined one.

So it is with all tales. They are transformative to the degree that they have become part of the greater tale. Only then is one's own story fully regained.

In past cultures this integration with a greater tale was guaranteed through the living body of myth. Through this body of myth everyone shared in the greater tales that birthed the culture of their birth. Greek mythology provided all the stories Greek men and women needed in order to orientate themselves to their world. The body of myth was an organic whole that not only informed the future but explained the past. All great myth provided an origin, a genesis that linked the present via the ancestors to the gods.

All this has been lost in our time. The body of myth that is our heritage has been largely stripped of its authority. The true myth of our time is the scientific world-view. It influences our civilization in the same way that the Greek myths influenced Greek culture. What this new myth does to us and to our relationship with all other stories is the important question that the tale of the Goose Girl addresses at the next level of interpretation.

At this level the story reveals its full meaning as a parable of humanity that traces the history of story from the remote past to the far future. Like many household tales, it is a kind of global myth, a story applicable everywhere and always. The trappings may be European, but the message is universal.

The Tale as a Parable of Humanity

At this level of interpretation we begin to see the hologram of meaning of which all other interpretations are merely pictures reflected in the shards. Through the Goose Girl we see deeply into the loss of story. The false maid stands for the powers of the intellect that obscure the reality of myth. Hiding behind the many masks of the modern mind, the maid robs Princess Story of her royal rights, her sacred past. Through cunning, the maid severs the princess from the old queen — the ancient Mother of Myth — the great giver of all 'the costly vessels of silver and gold and trinkets of gold and silver, and cups and jewels,' of horses that speak and handkerchiefs that carry the power of blood.

But the waiting-maid is also one of the gifts of the Mother, bestowed by the queenly wisdom of the past. She is part of the dowry; the catalyst for the alchemical process of the tale.

The maid's power unfolds in stages: first she refuses to serve. In her pride she will not step down from the 'high horse' of her pretensions. She abandons her duty as maid, her task as water bearer, servant of wisdom. Her refusal forces the princess to the ground. The princess loses her royal composure and with it the magical protection of the past: the white handkerchief with the three drops of blood. This is her first step into the initiations of loss. The second is the exchange of her royal garments of wisdom for the dress of the maid — the rags of the intellect. Then she loses her horse, the steady trustworthy voice of her intuition, and with it the last witness to her true identity.

At last the princess is forced to swear an oath of silence and self-denial. This is the most brilliant device of the maid, the most cunning of her schemes, for every myth, story and legend ever since has sworn that same oath: they have all succumbed to silence, agreed to deny their own reality, their true supremacy over the intellect. All stories have ceased to assert their true origin. Bound by their oath of silence they have become no more than mere fancy, children's fare, imaginations of the untutored mind, just a story; at most, collective projections or naive attempts to make meaning.

All myth has been usurped by the intellect. The maid has become the princess; the princess the maid. The plan has worked: story has lost her powers and the intellect sits on the throne.

The waiting-maid now mounts Falada, and the true bride the bad horse, and thus they enter the royal palace. There are great rejoicings over her arrival, and the prince springs forward to lift the waiting-maid from her horse, thinking she is his consort. The maid is conducted upstairs while the real princess is left standing below.

The rejoicing at court reflects the euphoria with which western society hails the advances of science and technology. Supported by mathematical proofs and a promising offspring of machinery and electronic wizardry, the reign of reason seems secure. The intellect rules supreme in the high court of truth. Its verdicts are convincing and its pronouncements are unquestioned.

Old Stories for a New Tale

In The Goose Girl, the old stories are exchanged for a new tale. Imagination is supplanted by the intellect as the wisdom of myths gives way to the clever concoctions of scientific theory. The purpose of the intellect, like that of the maid, is initially one of service. Each is there to serve the truth, to be a handmaiden of wisdom. Problems arise when the intellect claims dominance over imagination; when the maid usurps the princess; when the intellect's tale insists it is the only story.

For the intellect is the worst of storytellers. This is not surprising as its sole mission is to stick to the facts and discover the laws they contain, no more. When intellect builds a machine, it applies these laws. When intellect explains the whole universe as a machine, it is creating a myth. Intellect is a storyteller that knows only one story and repeats it over and over again.

Like the maid, the intellect is not content with its role. To be a servant of truth is not enough. Simply explaining the facts does not satisfy its ambitions: it longs to do what myths have always done. Intellect wants to explain the world with its own tale and make its own stories rule supreme. Like the old stories, it wants to shape the future.

Like the waiting-maid, intellect wants to become the princess, the queen, the new Mother of Myth, the great maker of stories. To this end, the intellect dethrones the power of myth, obscures the realities of stories, dresses them in the rags of analysis and interpretation, forces them into self-denial, and declares them useless before the law court of science.

Then the old king looked out of the window and saw her

standing in the courtyard, and noticed how dainty and delicate and beautiful she was, and instantly went to the royal apartment, and asked the bride about the girl she had with her who was standing down below in the courtyard, and who she was. I picked her up on my way for a companion, give the girl something to work at, that she may not stand idle.

But the old king had no work for her, and knew of none, so he said, I have a little boy who tends the geese, she may help him.

Divested of her powers, Princess Story is fit only to keep the company of geese, the most obstinate of birds. According to the maid, all stories but hers are stupid and only the obstinately backward cling to their truth.

The maid succeeds. The court of this world is blinded by her show of appearance. Society takes her stories for reality and demotes all other stories as fancy; her science fiction becomes science and her conclusions conclusive facts. The maid's unsupported assertions are accepted as truth. She is a genius of intrigue: she knows how to apply the right methods for the wrong purposes and how to cunningly arrange a minor truth to support major lies.

The story of the Goose Girl is explicitly precise about this strategy of deception. It is a fact that one of the young women who arrives at the court wears the garment of a princess. It is also a fact that the other wears a servant's dress. And it is true that one states that she is the princess while the other says nothing to the contrary. All this is apparently true, but it is not the truth.

Obvious truths can always be arranged for less obvious purposes. The maid is convincing because she has arranged the facts to match her tale. But it is not just her tale. Like Oedipus, she is only seemingly in charge of the situation. Her power is temporal. She is oblivious to the greater tale that has arranged her among the facts.

7. The Myths of the Intellect

Like many other popular fairytales, The Goose Girl reflects the death and resurrection of the imagination. The treacherous Loki is there behind the mask of the maid and the beautiful Baldur is the princess. The Goose Girl deals with the death of the imagination from the perspective of story itself. Its very theme is the usurping of story. To fully understand how stories can be usurped we need to turn to contemporary myth, to the very myth that has supplanted all other stories: the myth the intellect has created under the guise of science.

This is not to say that there is anything wrong with science itself. Science crowns the human search for truth. Objective science is the indispensable tool for both inner and outer progress. The method of science is one of the major achievements of western culture. But objective science is one thing, while science as a cover up for the myth-making of the intellect is another. It is the story-making of the intellect that needs to be examined. For its myths have usurped not only the older tales but also the story that science would otherwise tell.

Today, the intellect has become the only myth maker: thoughts that have become hypotheses that have become theories that have become truths that have become factual realities. A few philosophical minds may be aware that the only thing that science knows for certain is that *all* its present theories will be obsolete in fifty or a hundred years. But the intellect that is aware of its shortcomings is still the intellect. One may know one's limitations and still be limited by them. The labyrinth of the modern mind is a convoluted thing.

The complex powers of the intellect and its myths are not easily disentangled. They are part of a greater tale that is still being told — contemporary myth. And like all myths, they run deeper than thought. They are a second skin, tailored by world destiny.

The Myths of the Maid

The scientific myths created by the intellect are not restricted to those who practise or study them. They are omnipresent, and most potent in disguise. Without our knowing it, they colour the way we see the world. Our modern myths have paled the stars, eclipsed the sun and reduced the soul. They govern politics and shape history, they determine economics and influence education. They fuel conflicts between nations and give licence to cruelty. They are the tales that teach us to violate nature and exploit the world without regard for the future.

But they are all tales, not the truth. They are the maid's tale. They bear her imprint and the trademark of her method: that cunning arrangement of minor truths to support major lies, the skilful deception that substitutes the maid for the princess — *a reversal that turns truth into its opposite*.

What the maid does, so the intellect does too. It faithfully follows her example. She sets the precedent and it proceeds in her wake. Intellect always tells the same tale and it always resembles hers.

Take the theory of evolution. Evolution is a fact. But its theory is not. It is a myth constructed by the maid and bears her mark in every detail.

That fish precede amphibians and amphibians reptiles and reptiles mammals and mammals the human being is a great discovery made by a willing maid.

From the framework of this insight we can see deeply into the workings of Nature and watch her labour through the ages and give birth to ever more elaborate organisms. Her revelations in time and their tender echoes in the transitions in the developing embryo are among the most inspiring elements in the script of nature.

The rest is a tale told by the intellect and the usurping maid. And not a very original one: the plot is mere plagiarism. Darwin took it from the competitive economics of early industrialization and the science of his age. He squeezed the abundant revelations of nature into the tight corsets of the Victorian mind. He fitted his great discovery of evolution into a poor and constraining tale that exchanged the splendid garb of nature for the rags of his time. It is a tale that says little about nature, but much about the nature of the intellect.

Not surprisingly, the intellect is easily convinced by its own tale — it looked into a mirror and saw its own face. Like the fairytale stepmother, it preferred this tale above all others because it was its own offspring.

The idea of evolution was not entirely new. To the great myths of the past it was no stranger. These stories kept their ears to the utterances of the gods, listening for the first songs, for stories as old as memory and as ancient as time — creation myths.

Creation Myths

Creation myths have remained close to the Mother of Myth. They are
her first-born and contain her own account of her labour. Creation myths
are revelations of a divine ecology in which the destiny of the gods, the
manifestations of nature, and the biography of humanity are not separate
stories, but one great tale told in various fashions by various peoples.

For all its many variations, the essence of the creation myth is always
the same: all (except one!) share one fundamental trait. They trace the
biography of the world back to the gods, divinities, archetypes and
ancestral beings — from the great goddess Gaia birthing the generations of gods, to the giant Ymir of Nordic myth. In Mexican myth it is
Mother Growth, in American-Indian the Spider Woman; in Hebrew the
Elohim, in Finnish Ilmatar, the Mother of the Waters, labouring in the
first of seas.

Creation myths are primarily symbolic. Unconcerned with detail,
their focus is on cause rather than effect, intent rather than outcome,
process rather than result.

In the Indian creation myth the god Vishnu lies motionless on the
thousand-headed cobra of eternity. After he has created Brahma and
Brahma has created the world, Vishnu descends again and again into the
dense world of manifestations, ennobling, healing and furthering creation through his presence:

> Whenever justice and order are in danger, I come down and
> take shape.

In the Hindu tradition the incarnation of a divine being is called an
Avatar. According to a popular version of Indian creation myth, Vishnu
first took shape as a fish Avatar, then as a tortoise Avatar bearing the
whole world on its back, then the boar Avatar that rescues the earth. The
next incarnation is the fierce half-man, half-lion Avatar, then the dwarf
Avatar Vamana, then Purusha, the hunchbacked axeman and primordial
ascetic. Finally, Vishnu appears in perfected human form in the two
greatest of Indian heroes: Rama and Krishna.

Conceiving of Vishnu incarnating first as fish then reptile then mam-
mal then finally human forms, Indian wisdom conforms to the stages of
evolution millennia before evolutionary theory. But in all other respects
the old and the new myth are exactly opposite. They deal with the same

facts, but interpret them in diametrically different ways. The intellect's myth of evolution bears the mark of the maid in every detail. It tells the exact opposite tale of all other creation stories, and completely reverses the messages left by the Mother of Myth.

The divine creators are abandoned for dull matter; the conscious intent of primordial beings is discarded for unconscious accident, and the divinely guided process of evolution for unintentional mutation. Finally, the sacrificial love of the descending god as the incentive of evolution makes way for the universal mechanisms of hate: competition and the survival of the fittest, the biological equivalent of the war of everyone against everyone else.

Nothing in this myth is new. It is the same old tale that has been told in numerous myths, only here the names are changed and the meanings reversed. All positives have turned into negatives, and the initiatory power of love has been exchanged for the push and shove of hate.

The princess is silent and the eloquent maid cunningly arranges the proofs by turning the final effects of evolution — the physical world and its laws — into first causes. The intellect can do no other for this is the only story it knows. No new facts will change this tale, no new discovery alter its outcome; it will be told over and over again.

No matter how well the intellect equips itself with telescopes and microscopes, no matter how far it probes the depths of space and substance, it cannot escape its own limitations. It can only measure its own depth. However far the intellect projects theories into the past and future, the story will not change. It will always be the same pattern made in the mould of the maid: a pattern that reduces the glorious epic of the past to the mundane prose of the present; the artwork of this world to meaningless accidents in the probabilities of eternity; and the vast possibilities of the future to the fated theories of the present, to calculations provided by a calculating mind. In this story there is no purpose to the past and no point in the future; the present is unreal, the self an illusion.

In essence it is a marvellous, breathtaking enactment of myth. In one great crescendo we can watch the contemporary mind devouring itself, the suicide of meaning through meaning, the undoing of thought through thought. We can watch Nordic myth fulfil itself in the arena of mind, and the twilight of the intellect performed by the intellect itself.

The Great Deception

The myths the intellect creates under the pretence of science create the reality we know. Their verdict on the world is devastating; their judgement is harsh, their conclusions cruel. But their insights are not derived from reality, rather from their interpretation of it. They stem from the mind's preconceptions, and its deceptive orchestrations of truth in the service of the usurping maid, whose destiny matches the destiny of science and intellect — confronted with their own story they do not recognise it.

> When they had eaten and drunk, and were merry, the aged king asked the waiting-maid as a riddle, what punishment a person deserved who had behaved in such and such a way to her master, and at the same time related the whole story, and asked what sentence such a person merited. Then the false bride said, she deserves no better fate than to be stripped entirely naked, and put in a barrel which is studded inside with pointed nails, and two white horses should be harnessed to it, which will drag her along through one street after another, till she is dead.
>
> It is you, said the aged king, and you have pronounced your own sentence, and thus shall it be done unto you.

Just like the maid, the intellect produces dire judgements on its own creation. It condemns the picture of the world it has created and so condemns itself.

The so-called scientific world-view the intellect creates, let me repeat, is not the concern only of scientists. It is our shared reality, part of our contemporary myth. We all share in it. We live it, accept it, condemn ourselves through it, and suffer the judgements it makes.

At an unconscious level we are pained by a world that is accidental, by a life that has no meaning, by truths that are not true and a future that is doomed. We are made miserable by tales that condemn us to be cogs in a universal machine and pained by a world driven by the competition of everyone against everyone else.

Luckily it is only myth. Anti-myth. The maid's verdict on herself. The intellect's judgement on the facts it has selected to match its tale. Myth, nevertheless, that is part of our destiny and that we need to experience, suffer and overcome.

Unfortunately, we do not know this myth as a temporary stage of transition. We take it for real and lasting and so suffer the consequences. We believe in its nightmare and the nightmare comes true. If we could see the intellect's myth hiding within science, science would be freed to become the unobstructed instrument of truth, the handmaiden of wisdom, rather than a tool for a usurping storyteller. An ideal science would emancipate us from the compulsion of living out an unconscious myth.

Our mind is so used to the subliminal hopelessness of the myth that we hardly notice it any more. The soul suffers and like the princess it finds itself amid the ashes, in pain. But in this pain the true story is found and told. The true story breaks the power of the false maid and frees the princess from the silent acceptance of her fate.

The tale of the maid is pervasive. The myth of the intellect is only the tip of the iceberg. The maid's tale has infected more than our mind. It has frozen our soul. Below this tip of the iceberg it has pervaded our whole life. To thaw the soul from the cold spell of the intellect is one of the many tasks of story medicine. The tale of the Goose Girl helps us wake up to this spell, but it does not elaborate on the means by which it can be broken. It does not describe the procedures that break obsession and restore health. To study these, we need to visit *The Arabian Nights*.

8. *The Arabian Nights (1)*

The Arabian Nights is a collection of Persian tales. Their hero is Scheherazade, unofficial patron saint of story medicine. It is her marvellous telling of stories over one thousand and one nights that heals the fatal obsessions of King Sharya.

The stories of *The Arabian Nights* are ornamental and complicated like the patterns of Islamic art, aptly expressed in the flowing calligraphy of Arabic script rather than the staccato of western print. The tales are like a costly Persian rug, a flying carpet for the imagination woven from the weft and warp of stories within stories within stories.

In their original form they are adult tales, unsuitable for children, with moments of unashamed eroticism. Read superficially, they are simply entertainment, a noisy bazaar of tales. Read more closely, the labyrinth reveals itself as an authoritative manual on story medicine.

The Arabian Nights, a tale that contains so many other tales, is part of the great tale of transformation of ancient Iranian culture. No other culture has so thoroughly elaborated the contrast between good and evil and the part that the human being plays as an agent of transformation.

This theme is found in Iranian creation myth, where the Zurvan, God of Time, sacrifices for a thousand years in order to conceive a son. In fact, he creates two sons. When he doubts his own acts, he gives birth to his evil son Ahriman. From the merit of his sacrifices rises Ahura Mazda, God of Light.

In Persian myth, all creation results from the struggle between light and darkness. When Ahura Mazda creates the sheep, Ahriman creates the wolf. Creation is the interplay of dualities and the human being becomes the decisive factor in the transformation of evil into good. Thus human beings tame the wolf and make it into the sheepdog. The devourer of sheep becomes their protector and the enemy of shepherds becomes their most trusted friend.

This theme of transformation is omnipresent in Persian myth. We meet it when King Hushang overcomes fear through courage and sparks the first fire from flint. We meet it when King Djemshid, inspired by a nightly vision, makes his sword into a ploughshare. Transformation is the golden thread that links the ancient revelations of Zarathustra with

the teachings of Mani, and the mystic Sufism of Rumi with the content
of *The Arabian Nights.*

The Arabian Nights is the quintessence of story medicine, the epic of
the healing tale. Rightly read it reveals the archetypal pattern of obsession and the means of its healing:

> May the legends of the men of old be lessons to the people of
> our time so that a man may see those things which befell oth-
> ers beside himself: then he will honour and consider carefully
> the words and adventures of past people and derive benefit
> from it.
>
> May glory forever follow him who preserved the tales of
> our ancestors to be a guide to those who follow and who come
> after them.
>
> Now it is from among these very lessons that the stories
> called one thousand and one nights are taken together with all
> they contain of marvels and instruction.
>
> *From the introduction to The Thousand and One Nights*

Scheherazade and The Thousand and One Nights

The Arabian Nights tells the story of two brothers, King Sharya and
King Shazaman, both much loved by their people. When both were at
the height of their prosperous reigns, the older brother, Sharya, sent his
wazir to invite Shazaman to his court. Shazaman immediately set off
to visit his beloved brother, but had not gone far when he realized that
he had left something behind. He returned to his palace to find his wife
in the embrace of a slave. Enraged, he drew his sword and killed them
both.

Broken-hearted, Shazaman sets off again and arrives at his brother's
city with his face veiled in grief. He admits to his brother that he is
'stricken in the heart of his heart,' but does not disclose the cause of his
pain. When on the next day Sharya rides out to hunt, Shazaman remains
in the palace and stares through a window in his grief.

> While he was thus absorbed in grief, a secret gate of the sul-
> tan's palace suddenly opened, and there came out of it twenty
> women, in the midst of whom the queen was distinguished by

her majestic air. This princess, thinking that the king of Tartary
was gone a-hunting with his brother the sultan, came with her
retinue near the windows of his apartment.

He observed that the persons who accompanied the sultana
threw off their veils and long robes, that they might be more
at their ease, but he was greatly surprised to find that ten of
them were men, and that each of these took his mistress. The
sultana, on her part, was not long without her gallant. She
clapped her hands, and called 'Masoud, Masoud,' and immediately a man descended from a tree and ran towards her with
great speed.

Modesty will not allow, nor is it necessary, to relate what
passed between them. It is sufficient to say, that Shazaman saw
enough to convince him that his brother was as much to be
pitied as himself.

'How little reason had I,' said he, 'to think that none was so
unfortunate as myself? It is surely the unavoidable fate of all
husbands, since even the sultan my brother, who is sovereign
of so many dominions, and the greatest prince of the earth,
could not escape. What a fool am I to kill myself with grief.'

When suppertime came, they brought him the trays and he
ate with voracious appetite.

When Sharya returns and sees Shazaman in good spirits again, he asks
him for an explanation. Shazaman tells him of his own plight with his
wife and how his pain was relieved by witnessing the so much greater
misfortune of his brother. Sharya is shocked, but is convinced the next
day after becoming a witness himself.

'Oh heavens!' he exclaimed, 'what indignity! What horror!
Can the wife of a sovereign be capable of such infamous
conduct? After this, let no prince boast of being perfectly
happy. Alas! My brother,' continued he, embracing the king of
Tartary, 'let us both renounce the world. Honour is banished
out of it; if it flatter us one day, it betrays us the next. Let us
abandon our dominions, and go into foreign countries, where
we may lead an obscure life, and conceal our misfortunes.'
Shazaman did not at all approve of this plan, but did not
think fit to contradict Sharya in the heat of his passion. 'Dear

brother,' he replied, 'your will shall be mine. I am ready to follow you wherever you please: but promise me that you will return if we meet with anyone more unhappy than ourselves.' 'To this I agree,' said the sultan, 'but doubt much whether we shall.' 'I am not of your opinion in this,' replied the king of Tartary; 'I fancy our journey will be but short.'

The brothers leave the palace and travel until they come to a lonely tree near the salt sea.

There they rest until they see a cloud of black smoke approaching. Afraid, they climb into the tree. The smoke soon changes into a djinn, or genie, a demon of gigantic size carrying a box on his head. Ignorant of the two brothers hiding in the branches, the demon opened the box and released a beautiful young woman. Then he laid his head on her knees and fell asleep.

When the girl spies the two brothers in the treetops, she lifts the demon's head carefully from her knees and signs to the brothers to come down and make love to her. The kings are reluctant, but by threatening to waken the demon, she forces Shazaman and Sharya to do her will.

> At first they rejected it, but she obliged them to comply by her threats. Having obtained what she desired, she perceived that each of them had a ring on his finger, which she demanded. As soon as she had received them, she pulled out a string of other rings, which she showed the princes, and asked them if they knew what those jewels meant. 'No,' said they, 'we hope you will be pleased to inform us.' 'These are,' she replied, 'the rings of all the men to whom I have granted my favours. There are fourscore and eighteen, which I keep as memorials of them; and I asked for yours to make up the hundred. So I have had a hundred gallants already, notwithstanding the vigilance of this wicked genie, who never leaves me. He may lock me up in this glass box and hide me in the bottom of the sea, but I find methods to elude his vigilance. You may see by this, that when a woman has formed a project, there is no husband or lover that can prevent her from putting it in execution. Men had better not put their wives under such restraint, as it only serves to teach them cunning.' Having spoken thus to them, she put their rings on the same string with the rest, and sitting

down by the monster, as before, laid his head again upon her lap, and made a sign to the princes to depart.

They returned immediately the way they had come, and when they were out of sight of the lady and the genie, Sharya said to Shazaman, 'Well, brother, what do you think of this adventure? Has not the genie a very faithful mistress? And do you not agree that there is no wickedness equal to that of women?' 'Yes, brother,' answered the king of Great Tartary; 'and you must also agree that the monster is more unfortunate, and more to be pitied than ourselves. Therefore, since we have found what we sought for, let us return to our dominions, and let not this hinder us from marrying. For my part, I know a method by which to preserve the fidelity of my wife inviolable. I will say no more at present, but you will hear of it in a little time, and I am sure you will follow my example.

Text of Dr Jonathan Scott

When King Sharya returned to his city he had all his wives and slaves put to death. Then he ordered his wazir to bring him every night a young virgin, whom he ravished and on the next morning had slain. This continued until there were no virgins left, except the wazir's own daughters.

The Wazir had two daughters, Sharazad and Dunyazad, of whom the elder had perused the books, annals and legends of preceding kings, and the stories, examples and instances of bygone men and things; indeed it was said that she had col- lected a thousand books of histories relating to antique races and departed rulers. She had perused the works of the poets and knew them by heart; she had studied philosophy and the sciences, arts and accomplishments; and she was pleasant and polite, wise and witty, well read and well bred.

Trans. Sir Richard Burton

Scheherazade offers herself as a ransom. Her father is opposed to her plan, but in the end he gives in and Scheherazade is married to King Sharya.

The Nested Story and the Cliffhanger

On her wedding night Scheherazade begins to weave her complex web of stories. She continues night after night, always ending in a cliffhanger, which keeps the king longing for the rest of her tale. In order to hear the conclusion he spares her life, one night at a time.

From her first telling we meet two potent devices of story medicine: the cliffhanger and the nested story. Like a Russian babushka doll, the stories nest one in another, stories within stories within stories, to form a complicated organism that parallels the intricate patterns of Islamic ornamentation.

The nesting reflects the body of story, the greater tale that encompasses the smaller tales. The totality of tales and myth form a highly complicated organism. Greek myth too is no collection of separate tales, but an intrinsic body of stories that are related as intimately as the organs and functions of the human body.

Initially all stories, myths and tales were in continuous movement. Changing, shifting, growing, they were as alive as those who told them. Every story has multiple ways of expressing itself, reflecting the mobility of the archetypes. Only gradually do they condense and harden into the forms we know. Their last life is lost in script. Paper is their shroud, books their coffin.

Nested stories are a remnant of this organic life. They resist the intellect and its compulsive need of order and obsessive control. Even in print they resist being neatly sliced into separate parts. Nested stories preserve the motherhood of the imagination. They mirror the continuous creativity of the archetypal world and belong to the feminine aspect of spirituality that linear intellect lacks. It is this quality that makes them therapeutic for the rigid intellect and its close relative: obsession.

Obsessions too are contractions of soul. The vast expanses of inner life are reduced, condensed; instead of many stories there is only one story, told over and over again. The convoluted dynamics of Scheherazade's nested stories are an injection of life into the linear imprisonment of King Sharya's obsession.

The cliffhanger performs a similar function. A tale kept open-ended and alive does the same to the listener. It allows neither habitual ending nor foregone conclusions. A cliffhanger story always opens a space. It teaches the listener how to listen, to remain open, to expect more, to have patience, to look forward to the unknown. It keeps the soul suspended in a healthy mood of expectation and it counteracts the desire for control. The open-ended story is a great teacher of process, and offers initiation into the gifts of time.

The Soul's Story

Scheherazade is a genius of story medicine. She knows how to tell the right story at the right time. She weaves a story carpet that never ends. She knows when to stop a tale and when to leave it open. She understands the picture language of the soul and speaks it with eloquence. She administers her medicine consciously, carefully. Her tales are not arbitrary; they are carefully chosen to suit the ailing king. By means of her stories she initiates him into his own story.

Like Odysseus and Parzival, the king hears his own tale. But he does so unwittingly. He is not a hero like Odysseus, but a victim. He is not aware how much the stories reflect his own predicament.

Though he is a king and outwardly powerful, Sharya is inwardly helpless. Scheherazade's stories bypass his obsessed persona and speak to his depth, where they are recognised and act medicinally.

I have often encountered this phenomenon of depth-recognition. Most people have a favourite story, and without exception, this story reflects their major predicament in life. The soul recognises the medicine it needs and leans towards it.

The relationship between story and biography may be obvious to everyone but the subject, who is generally unable to see the connection. It is in the subject's blind spot, too close to be seen. The everyday personality is too enmeshed, too identified with the theme of the predicament — it almost *is* that theme. The predicament cannot be seen because everything is seen through it.

But the deep knower within knows the story and loves it. To the soul, the right story is like the light as it appears to someone walking in a dark tunnel. It engenders hope and shows a way forward.

Stories that are medicinal do not merely reflect problems, they integrate them into the greater totality of the tale. They put the problem in perspective, assign it its proper place as an incentive to development — a beginning rather than an ending, an opportunity rather than a pitfall.

We can learn the art of medicinal storytelling from Scheherazade. Already her first tale, of the Merchant and the Ifrit, has other tales nested in its fabric.

The Merchant and the Ifrit

A rich merchant rests on one of his journeys beneath a tree. He refreshes himself with a couple of dates and throws their stones away.

Suddenly an Ifrit, a demon, appears and tells the merchant that the stone he has carelessly thrown has killed one of his children. He brandishes his sword and is about to kill the innocent man but the merchant begs him in the name of Allah to give him time to settle his affairs. He promises the Ifrit he will then return and face death.

The demon is persuaded and the merchant does as he promised. He orders his affairs and returns on the appointed date to be beheaded by the Ifrit. While he is waiting for his executioner to appear, three sheiks pass by, one leading a gazelle, the second accompanied by two dogs and the third by a mule.

When the three travellers hear the pitiful tale of the merchant, they decide to stay with him in his last hour.

When the Ifrit appears brandishing his sword, the first sheik offers the demon a story in an exchange for one third of the merchant's blood. The Ifrit, like all demons, cannot resist a good story. He agrees to the bargain and the first sheik tells his tale.

The Merchant and the Ifrit is the opening of Scheherazade's tale and it relates directly to the situation at hand. The merchant who is to be beheaded for no apparent reason reflects Scheherazade's own position with the obsessed king: he plans to behead her the next morning.

The demon, however, is persuaded to grant more time, and so the story sets the precedent the king will soon follow. Scheherazade bargains for time by leaving her story unfinished, just as the three sheiks offer their stories as ransom for the merchant's life — a bargain the king can no more resist than the demon can.

Moreover, the stories told by the three sheiks relate directly to the obsession of the king: they touch on his wounds and leave a healing balm. They open the imaginative conversation between ailment and remedy.

Each story deals with unfaithfulness from a different angle. The first is about a gazelle, who was the first sheik's former wife and who plotted the death of his son and slave mother with cunning enchantments. The second tale is about two dogs who were brothers of the second sheik and abused his generosity and care. The third is about a mule, the former wife of the third sheik, who returned home unannounced to find his wife in the arms of a slave. Before he was able to act, his wife, who was also a sorceress, enchanted him into a dog and whipped him out of the house. Luckily his neighbour's daughter, who is also versed in magic, breaks the spells. She returns the sheik to human form and enchants the unfaithful wife into a mule.

The three stories build in intensity to the last which has obvious parallels with the story of King Sharya. The story touches the core of the king's ailment. He too found his wife unfaithful. In his obsession, he too was enchanted, and still is at this stage. Scheherazade's tales open the possibility of transformation, liberation, the end of enchantment and healing.

Scheherazade's image of enchantment vividly describes the impact of traumatic experiences. They enchant the many colours of the soul into one prevailing monochrome. Each hurt casts an unconscious spell that clouds our perception like darkly coloured glass. Our deepest wounds become the lenses through which we see the world. Like a magical telescope they always point us towards the same selection of painful experience on the rich and varied canvas of the soul.

But these stories are only the first opening, a beginning. Many more will have to be told before the king is healed.

9. *The Arabian Nights (2)*

To fully appreciate *The Thousand and One Nights* we need a key to unlock its depths. This key can be found in the user manual that most stories contain within them, often to be found close to the beginning. The tale of the Fisherman and the Djinn, which follows the tales of the three sheiks, holds the key to Scheherazade's treasure chambers, and I include here a substantial part of it.

The Fisherman and the Djinn

It has reached me, O auspicious King, that there was a fisherman well stricken in years who had a wife and three children, and withal was of poor condition. Now it was his custom to cast his net every day four times, and no more. On a day he went forth about noontide to the seashore, where he made a cast with his net and waited till it settled to the bottom. Then he gathered the cords together and hauled away at it, but found it weighty. And however much he drew it landward, he could not pull it up, so he carried the ends ashore and drove a stake into the ground and made the net fast to it. Then he stripped and dived into the water all about the net, and left not off working hard until he had brought it up.

He rejoiced thereat and, donning his clothes, went to the net, when he found in it a dead jackass which had torn the meshes. Now when he saw it, he exclaimed in his grief, 'There is no Majesty and there is no Might save in Allah the Glorious, the Great!

The fisherman, when he had looked at the dead ass, got it free of the net and wrung out and spread his net. Then he plunged into the sea, saying, 'In Allah's name!' and made a cast and pulled at it, but it grew heavy and settled down more firmly than the first time. Now he thought that there were fish in it, and he made it fast and, doffing his clothes, went into the water, and dived and hauled until he drew it up upon dry land.

Then found he in it a large earthen pitcher which was full of
sand and mud, and seeing this, he was greatly troubled.

So he prayed pardon of Allah and, throwing away the jar,
wrung his net and cleansed it and returned to the sea the third
time to cast his net, and waited till it had sunk. Then he pulled
at it and found therein potsherds and broken glass. Then, raising his eyes heavenward, he said: 'O my God! Verily Thou
knowest that I cast not my net each day save four times. The
third is done and as yet Thou hast vouchsafed me nothing. So
this time, O my God, deign give me my daily bread.'

Then, having called on Allah's name, he again threw his net
and waited its sinking and settling, whereupon he hauled at it
but could not draw it in for that it was entangled at the bottom.

Thereupon he stripped and, diving down to the net, busied
himself with it till it came to land. Then he opened the meshes
and found therein a cucumber-shaped jar of yellow copper,
evidently full of something, whose mouth was made fast with
a leaden cap stamped with the seal ring of our Lord Solomon,
son of David (Allah accept the twain!).

Seeing this, the fisherman rejoiced and said, 'If I sell it in
the brass bazaar, 'tis worth ten golden dinars.' He shook it and,
finding it heavy, continued: 'Would to Heaven I knew what is
herein. But I must and will open it and look to its contents and
store it in my bag and sell it in the brass market.' And taking
out a knife, he worked at the lead till he had loosened it from
the jar.

Presently there came forth from the jar a smoke which spired
heavenward into ether (whereat he again marvelled with mighty
marvel), and which trailed along earth's surface till presently,
having reached its full height, the thick vapour condensed, and
became an Ifrit huge of bulk, whose crest touched the clouds
while his feet were on the ground. His head was as a dome, his
hands like pitchforks, his legs long as masts, and his mouth big
as a cave. His teeth were like large stones, his nostrils ewers, his
eyes two lamps, and his look was fierce and lowering.

Now when the fisherman saw the Ifrit his teeth chattered,
his spittle dried up, and he became blind about what to do.
Upon this the Ifrit looked at him and cried, 'Be of good cheer,
O Fisherman!' Quoth the fisherman, 'Why biddest thou me to

be of good cheer?' And he replied, 'Because of thy having to die an ill death in this very hour.' Said the fisherman, 'Wherefore shouldest thou kill me, and what thing have I done to deserve death, I who freed thee from the jar, and saved thee from the depths of the sea, and brought thee up on the dry land?'

Replied the Ifrit, 'Ask of me only what mode of death thou wilt die, and by what manner of slaughter shall I slay thee.' Rejoined the fisherman, 'What is my crime, and wherefore such retribution?' Quoth the Ifrit, 'Hear my story, O Fisherman! Know that I am one among the heretical Djann, and I sinned against Solomon, David-son (on the twain be peace!)

'When Solomon bound me, he took refuge with Allah and bade me embrace the True Faith and obey his behests. But I refused, so, sending for this cucurbit, he shut me up therein and stopped it over with lead, whereon he impressed the Most High Name, and gave his orders to cast me into the midmost of the ocean.

'There I abode a hundred years, during which I said in my heart, "Whoso shall release me, him will I enrich forever and ever."

'But the full century went by and, when no one set me free, I entered upon the second fivescore saying, "Whoso shall release me, for him I will open the hoards of the earth."

'Still no one set me free, and thus four hundred years passed away. Then quoth I, "Whoso shall release me, for him will I fulfil three wishes." Yet no one set me free.

'Thereupon I waxed wroth with exceeding wrath and said to myself, "Whoso shall release me from this time forth, him will I slay, and I will give him choice of what death he will die." And now, as thou hast released me, I give thee full choice of deaths.'

The fisherman, hearing the words of the Ifrit, said, 'O Allah! Spare my life, so Allah spare thine, and slay me not, lest Allah set one to slay thee.' But the Ifrit replied, 'There is no help for it. Die thou must, so ask by way of boon what manner of death thou wilt die.'

Upon this the fisherman said to himself: 'This is a Djinn, and I am a man to whom Allah has given a passably cunning wit, so I will now cast about to compass his destruction by my contrivance and by mine intelligence, even as he took counsel only of his malice and his forwardness.'

He began by asking the Ifrit, 'Hast thou indeed resolved to kill me?' And, receiving for all answer, 'Even so,' he cried, 'In the name of Allah, if I question thee on a certain matter, wilt thou give me a true answer?' The Ifrit replied 'Yea,' but, hearing mention of the Most Great Name, his wits were troubled and he said with trembling, 'Ask and be brief.'

Quoth the fisherman: 'How didst thou fit into this bottle which would not hold thy hand — no, nor even thy foot — and how came it to be large enough to contain the whole of thee?' Replied the Ifrit, 'What! Dost not believe that I was all there?' And the fisherman rejoined, 'Nay! I will never believe it until I see thee inside with my own eyes.'

The Evil Spirit on the instant shook and became a vapour, which condensed and entered the jar little and little, till all was well inside, when lo! the fisherman in hot haste took the leaden cap with the seal and stoppered therewith the mouth of the *jar* and called out to the Ifrit, saying: 'By Allah, I will throw thee into the sea before us.' Now when the Ifrit heard this from the fisherman and saw himself in limbo, he was minded to escape, but this was prevented by Solomon's seal.

So he knew that the fisherman had outwitted him, and he waxed lowly and submissive and began humbly …

When the djinn realizes he is caught, he begs for mercy and promises riches. But the fisherman is not easily persuaded. He justifies his refusal to trust the genie with the tale of the ungrateful King Yunan, who killed his benefactor and so caused his own death. The tale of King Yunan ends with the fisherman's words to the genie:

'Now, O Ifrit,' continued the fisherman, 'know that if King Yunan had spared the sage, Duban, God had spared him; but he refused, and desired his destruction; therefore God destroyed him; and thou, O Ifrit, if thou hadst spared me, God had spared thee, and I had spared thee; but thou desiredst my death; therefore will I put thee to death imprisoned in this bottle, and will throw thee here into the sea.'

However, when the djinn promises not to harm the fisherman, but reward him with riches, the poor man is persuaded and releases the djinn again.

The story of King Yunan clearly has a medicinal effect on the genie; he stands by his word and spares the fisherman's life. As a reward for his liberation he leads the fisherman into an adventure in which he becomes instrumental in liberating a prince and his whole realm from cruel enchantment. This prince too had been enchanted by an unfaithful wife who betrayed him with a slave. When the prince harms the slave, she turns him into marble from the waist down and returns every day to torture his upper body with a whip. Then she covers his open wounds with a hair shirt to prolong his pain while she returns to care for her injured lover.

At this point in the tale, two motifs are brought powerfully together. The transformation of the demon — the bottled up genie — and the liberation of the enchanted and tortured prince — an Islamic variation on the wounded Grail King, Anfortas.

In fact they are the same motif, seen from different perspectives. The demon is an objectified part of the soul, perceived as an autonomous, outward reality. The tortures of the prince are the subjective experience of the demonic, 'bottled up' in the interior of the soul. Every obsession is a bottled up psychic power.

These paired motifs lead Sharya into the core of his pain. The young prince has suffered the same sexual wound. His is the imaginal replica of the king's suffering. The king has lost his power to combat his obsession. His will — that is, his lower part — is maimed, turned to stone. He can no longer move. At the same time he suffers immense and continuous pain at the hands of his wife who returns each day to torture him. When she covers his wounds with the cruel hair shirt, she mirrors what the king does to himself when he wraps one pain in another, when he prolongs his suffering by inflicting it outwardly on others, and ultimately on himself.

Through this story Sharya is confronted with the depth of his wounding and with the potential of healing. He is able to accept in imaginative form what he would have rejected in conceptual terms. He gains self-knowledge as Scheherazade unties the painful knots of his soul, carefully opening the bottle of his imprisonment.

The Fourfold Pattern of Soul Dynamics

The key to a deeper understanding of *The Arabian Nights* is contained in the story of the Fisherman and the Djinn. Again it has to be sought in the fine print of composition.

The first thing that strikes us is the recurrence of the number four. Four times the fisherman casts his net, and four times the imprisoned genie promises a reward. Each time the fisherman draws his net back from the sea the work is more tiresome and the catch more disappointing: a dead ass, a mudded earthen jar, broken pots and shards of glass.

At first the final catch seems fortunate, but it turns into a fatal threat: a djinn poised to annihilate the one who frees him.

The genie in turn tells his own tale of misery. It too unfolds in four stages. Long waiting to be freed, he initially vowed to reward his liberator with eternal riches, then with all the treasures of the earth and then with three wishes of the heart. When all this is to no avail, the desperate demon makes a fourth vow, to kill the one who sets him free.

The fourfold pattern in the Fisherman and the Ifrit parallels the stages of obsession. In the cover story of *The Arabian Nights* these four stages appear in the sequence of events that meets the two brothers, Sharya and Shazaman. The first is Shazaman's confrontation with his unfaithful wife. The second is his observation of Sharya's even greater misfortune. The third is the two brothers' encounter with the young girl captured by the djinn, and the fourth is Sharya's own pattern of consummation and death, the pattern that Scheherazade is trying to break.

If we look at this tale as an in-depth study of soul dynamics, it can initiate us into the fourfold pattern of obsession and its healing.

The first stage is that of *witness*. Confronted with his wife's unfaithfulness, Shazaman is still able to respond. He takes the action required by the custom of the day and feels appropriate pain.

In the second stage he has lost his will to act. He is a mere observer and even finds relief from his pain by watching the greater misfortunes of his brother. (The story artfully uses two brothers in order to elaborate on the unconscious details that accompany the soul's journey into obsession.)

> When Shah-Zeman beheld this spectacle he said within himself, By Allah! My affliction is lighter than this! His vexation

and grief were alleviated, and he no longer abstained from
sufficient food and drink.

Trans. Edward William Lane

By merely observing the betrayal in his brother's house Shazaman
indirectly and unconsciously consents to what he sees, a point further
emphasized by the release he derives from it. I call this the stage of *consent*, albeit that it is unconscious.

The third stage is the meeting of the two brothers with the Ifrit and the
young girl captured in the case. This is the stage of the *accomplice* and
it follows by necessity that of unconscious consent. The two kings are
forced to commit the same kind of betrayal that they have suffered. They
have little choice. Freedom is increasingly diminished in the downward
spiral of obsession, a dynamic in which pain is released with greater pain
and hopelessness with despair.

> When the two kings heard these words from her lips they were
> struck with the utmost astonishment, and said, one to the other,
> 'If this is an Ifrit, and a greater calamity has happened unto
> him than that which has befallen us, this is a circumstance
> that should console us' — and immediately they departed, and
> returned to the city.

The story portrays the vicious circle of negative intensity, the tight-
ening noose of obsession, the shrinking of freedom to the point of
despair.

The fourth and final stage is that of *perpetrator*. Here the sufferer has
become the one who inflicts the suffering. The king's disappointment
with love becomes his appointment with hate. He numbs his pain by
inflicting it on others. He covers his wound with the bandage of cruelty
and hides his helplessness behind the illusion of power.

Sharya is sucked into the demonic whirlpool of despair where pain
eternally propagates itself in vicious cycles of destruction. This stage
differs from the third because of the active part the perpetrator plays;
the accomplice is still somewhat reluctant. The acts of the perpetrator
have their origin within. Outward incentives have turned into inward
compulsions.

A Thousand and One Nightmares

Sharya's tale is true in the way that all stories are true: it may never have happened in a particular time and place, but it is always happening everywhere.

And it has never happened more intensely than in our time. For we have the means to multiply Sharya's vicious cycle of obsession and administer it to any one at any time. We have made his destiny a lifestyle. The bitter pill of his story has become the staple tale of our time.

Most children in the western world enact the fourfold ritual of derangement on a daily basis, leaning comfortably back on the family sofa while watching multiple murders on the TV screen: blood spilling, cars exploding, women being raped. Imagine a child actually seeing people mowed down by machine gun, or the intimate details of sex.

In real life any incident remotely like this would evoke intense reaction. Nobody would stand by watching a human being killed or violated.

The moment a child watches violence without reaction, emotion, fear, shock, disgust or revulsion it has taken the step from witness to consent. That child has slipped into Sharya's shoes.

To watch violence without reaction is to silently agree to it. To be comfortable with brutality and to remain at ease in its presence is to unconsciously consent to it. In this moment the child begins to take cruelty for entertainment, crime for what is permissible and rape for normal.

This happens so fast that one step stumbles into the next. The stage of consent turns into that of unconscious accomplice as violence becomes entertainment and the watching of cruelty becomes a source of pleasure.

The average American has seen some 30,000 murders on TV by the age of seventeen. Witnessed the first, consented to the next and actively sought the rest. Girls and boys have been made accomplice by a mixture of common consent, ignorance and neglect and by the mindless doing of what everyone does. In the great quantum sleep of the technological age the slaughter of innocence is enacted in every house.

While TV takes the child from witness to accomplice, computer games prepare the perpetrator. These are every child's chance to actively crush, kill, shoot, bomb, terrorize, drown and explode with abandon and full attention to the details of destruction. Here is the electronic training ground for all possible means of death, an unmatched opportunity to fight, conquer and kill until the last remnant of sensitivity is purged from the soul. This is the stage of virtual perpetrator, the happy murderer, the ecstatic destroyer.

In the depth memory of the soul nothing is lost. Under hypnosis every movie ever watched can be recalled in great detail. Every act of violence, every murder, every rape remains etched on the soul's interior skin.

Some individuals may be immune to the impact of media indoctrination. Some may be able to come to terms with the pervading anti-myth and its constant enactment on the public screen. Even children may be able to resist the assault with the loving help of a parent.

But we are dealing with a pervasive myth, and if we do not change it, it will change us. It took many hundreds of years to turn the dynamics of Oedipus' destiny into the philosophy of Socrates, and millennia for Egypt to lie down in the tombs its myth had prepared. Myth is fulfilled over time. The process is slow but steady. The changes are imperceptible at first. Often they are only obvious in hindsight.

This did not matter with the largely wholesome myths of the past. But it matters very much now. The new myths are of our making and they shape our reality just as ancient myths shaped earlier realities. What at present is only a pastime for a child, a mind-game for a teenager and entertainment for an adult is fast becoming a way of life. Nightmares can become reality, particularly if they are continuously reinforced through ritual.

Rituals might be considered condensed myths, regularly enacted to ensure their impact. The Jewish Sabbath, for instance, is the weekly celebration of a decisive moment that shaped the destiny of the people of Israel — the end of slavery in Egypt and the beginning of their home-coming. The Christian mass is a remembrance of the essential deeds of Christ. The Moslem pilgrimage to Mecca recalls a crucial episode in Mohammed's life.

But the ritual of religious myths pales against the ritual of regular media use. In the end it is not what we believe in but what we spend time with. For what we spend time with is what we really believe in.

Our daily rituals may not appear to affect our soul immediately. But they will do so over time as they change the culture we live in. To keep them in check we need to monitor the impact contemporary myth and media have on our life, particularly on the life of children.

The Imagination at Risk

The content of the media is only one part of the problem. Another is the act of engagement with the media itself. Television, videos and computer games are largely image-based. This makes them technological equivalents or substitutes for the imagination itself. Children who are overexposed to these media will fail to develop their imagination.

This is even more harmful than the effect of the content they take in. While the content remains somewhat external, the imagination is a crucial inner capacity with whose help we define and constantly reinvent ourselves. It is our most essential tool of self-development. Our authentic ideas and deeds have their origin in this capacity.

The whole edifice of our culture is a result of applied imagination. All major breakthroughs in science are the result of imagination, and so is every invention. Our complex technology is entirely a brainchild of the imagination, as are all the productions of art.

The imagination is a capacity central to being human. It is a form of inner activity through which we create our own pictures, visions, ideas and plans. Childhood is the cradle of this activity and like all capacities it can flourish or its development can be stunted. The imagination develops through continuous and active use, through unimpeded picture making unfolding in childhood fancy. The imagination is a vital element of the soul. If it is not properly used it atrophies.

It is this picture making that is suppressed by the visual media. Passive reception is substituted for inner activity. The tender opening of the mind's eye is overpowered by the glaring screen and authentic picture making is overtaken by prefabricated images.

The difference between a passive and an active imagination is exemplified by Sharya and Scheherazade. The king's obsession is not just a result of his disappointment with women. The unfolding events only provided the means for the disposition of his soul to become apparent. His obsession is equally due to his inability to come to terms with the events in his life, his inability to see things differently and find meaning in his pain. Obsessions always have a fixed content. They are patterns of thoughts, pictures and feelings that cannot be changed.

Sharya has lost the capacity for inner movement, the power to see things in a different light. He lacks active imagination. Only the imagination can change our response, find new meaning in an old and painful tale and transform the way we respond. It is this absence of inner activity that makes Sharya fall prey to his obsession. He has lost the power to navigate the ship of his soul. He is helpless against his story and the pictures that plague him.

So it is with a child who is helpless against the hypnotic power of TV. The prefabricated images act in exactly the same way on the child as Sharya's obsession works on him. Both overwhelm the soul and carry it helplessly along.

The result is a victim. Someone who has no choice. The mark of his soul-life is passivity. A victim may react, but not act. The opposite of the victim is the hero. Heroes act constructively. They do not remain spellbound by events. They use their imagination to change and transform whatever situation they meet.

Scheherazade is the active hero of *The Arabian Nights*. It is her imagination that makes her the heroine we love. Everyone else falls victim to the king's obsession. Nobody else knows how to remedy the situation. Nobody else has the idea, the foresight, the vision of how to proceed. It takes imagination to see the possibility of healing where others see none, imagination to devise the long-term strategy of one thousand and one nights and imagination to determine the right tale for the right moment.

Sharya exemplifies the pattern of the victim. Scheherazade shows the steps the hero takes by means of the imagination.

Scheherazade's Ladder of Love

Scheherazade confronts Sharya's demonic obsession with imaginative means. Her stories work like a homeopathic dilution in which obsession is reduced to its pure essence, its dynamic action. In this state the medicine is understood not by the intellect, but by the deeper layers of soul, where the essence of the story speaks to the essence of the human being. story medicine thus begins to cure not the symptoms, but the actual cause of the suffering.

True healing is a process that takes time and care. One treatment is not enough, one story not sufficient. Many more have to follow to break the old pattern and build the new. Scheherazade, of course, is well prepared for this. She is graced with an abundant body of story.

She had read various books of histories, and the lives of preceding kings, and stories of past generations: it is asserted that she had collected together a thousand books of histories, relating to preceding generations and kings, and works of the poets.

Scheherazade doesn't just know stories, she embodies the power of the imagination and uses it for the situation at hand. She is able to live what she preaches. Her deeds tell the story of her heart, a story that, in its stages, parallels the king's, except that her story is conscious and his is not.

The king's story reveals the four stages of obsession. It is the tale of the intellect uninformed by soul, of masculine mind without the benefit of feminine imagination.

Scheherazade's behaviour illustrates the stages of ascending health, the tale of the imaginative soul, the four major acts of integration on the ladder of love. Climbing this ladder, she reverses the stages of obsession into their opposites.

She, like the king, encounters the stage of *witness*. He was confronted with the unfaithfulness of his wife; Scheherazade with the king's cruelty and obsession. But, unlike the king, Scheherazade is not caught in obsession's lure. Using her imagination she counteracts his reactive hate with her active love, and his disappointment with hope.

In stage two, she counters his unconscious consent with her conscious *sacrifice*, offering herself as a ransom for the daughters of the Musselmans and to effect their delivery out of the hands of the king. What has lamed and brutalized him has stirred her into the highest form of action: sacrifice.

In the third stage, she reverses the helplessness of the unwilling accomplice into the transformative work of the healer. With the help of story she brings change. She accomplishes *transformation*.

Through her long and conscious work she finally liberates the king. She leads him from the isolated confines of obsession into communion with story, meaning, and herself. Death becomes life, hatred love and the pattern of sickness is replaced with a story of health.

The final tale in *The Arabian Nights* is the story of tender and innocent love. It crowns the body of stories with the diadem of love. The king is healed, the kingdom saved. Sharya marries Scheherazade. She, who has communicated her soul, now is in *communion* with him.

From desperate beginnings Scheherazade has led him on the long road of story medicine. She has shown him his own condition in the mirror of tales, taken his soul by the hand into the realm of story, picture, and imagination. She has brought colour to the monochrome of his soul, imaginative diversity to the monotony of his mind, and humour to his solitary gloom. She has brought a whole world of stories to his singular tale of betrayal. She has rebuilt his body of story and so wrought healing.

The Arabian Nights initiates us into the depths of soul. The sequence lays bare the structure of obsession and the fourfold ladder of descent. Such structures are not premeditated. They are not superimposed on story. Like all true art they arise spontaneously from the matrix of what is universally human.

Sharya is a picture of the masculine psyche, the intellect-driven mind that can be found in both men and women. His destiny is symptomatic of the modern human being, *homo intellectus*, of western society and much of present day civilization. Like many of our contemporaries, Sharya had lost contact with soul, with the feminine in himself, with imagination and the realm of story. He is healed by an abundance of story medicine, story after story, night after night, until his imagination is restored.

Imagination is the feminine complement to the masculine intellect. She is the true bride. Her resurrection brings healing to the king. She bestows on him what he lacks: the ladder of story on which he may climb from the lowest levels of his obsessive state to the highest manifestation of love that is the final story of *The Arabian Nights.*

10. The Art of the New Scheherazade

The story cycle of *The Arabian Nights* reveals the stages of healing in the life of King Sharya. It also reveals the attitude of the true healer, one that is fundamentally different from the attitude of the king as well as everyone else. It is the attitude we need if we want to bring about change. But we can only acquire it if we change ourselves and the way we view the world.

How such a change can come about is best illustrated by a Native American tale, the story of Jumping Mouse.

The Story of Jumping Mouse

Once there was a mouse. He was a busy mouse, searching everywhere, touching his whiskers to the grass and looking. He was busy as all mice are, busy with mice things. But once in a while he would hear an odd sound. He would lift his head, squinting hard to see, his whiskers wiggling in the air, and he would wonder. One day he scurried up to a fellow mouse and asked him, 'Do you hear a roaring in your ears, my brother?'

'No, no,' answered the other mouse, not lifting his busy nose from the ground. 'I hear nothing. I am busy now. Talk to me later.'

He asked another mouse the same question and the mouse looked at him strangely. 'Are you foolish in your head? What sound?' he asked and slipped into a hole in a fallen cotton-wood tree.

The little mouse shrugged his whiskers and busied himself again, determined to forget the whole matter. But there was that roaring again. It was faint, very faint, but it was there! One day, he decided to investigate the sound just a little. Leaving the other busy mice, he scurried a little way away and listened again. There it was! He was listening hard when suddenly, someone said hello.

'Hello little brother,' the voice said, and mouse almost

jumped right out of his skin. He arched his back and tail and was about to run.

'Hello,' again said the voice. 'It is I, brother raccoon.' And sure enough, it was! 'What are you doing here all by yourself, little brother?' asked the raccoon. The mouse blushed, and put his nose almost to the ground. 'I hear a roaring in my ears and I am investigating it,' he answered timidly.

'A roaring in your ears?' replied the raccoon as he sat down with him. 'What you hear, little brother, is the river.'

'The river?' mouse asked curiously. 'What is a river?'

'Walk with me and I will show you the river,' raccoon said.

Little mouse was terribly afraid, but he was determined to find out once and for all about the roaring. 'I can return to my work,' he thought, 'after this thing is settled, and possibly this thing may aid me in all my busy examining and collecting. And my brothers all said it was nothing. I will show them. I will ask raccoon to return with me and I will have proof.'

'All right raccoon, my brother,' said mouse, 'lead on to the river. I will walk with you.'

Little mouse walked with raccoon. His little heart was pounding in his breast. The raccoon was taking him upon strange paths and little mouse smelled the scent of many things that had gone by his way. Many times he became so frightened he almost turned back. Finally, they came to the river! It was huge and breathtaking, deep and clear in places, and murky in others. Little mouse was unable to see across it because it was so great. It roared, sang, cried, and thundered on its course. Little mouse saw great and little pieces of the world carried along on its surface.

'It is powerful!' little mouse said, fumbling for words.

'It is a great thing,' answered the raccoon, 'But here, let me introduce you to a friend.'

In a smoother, shallower place was a lily pad, bright and green. Sitting upon it was a frog, almost as green as the pad it sat on. The frog's white belly stood out clearly.

'Hello, little brother,' said the frog. 'Welcome to the river.'

'I must leave you now,' cut in raccoon, 'but do not fear, little brother, for frog will care for you now.' And raccoon left, looking along the river bank for food that he might wash and eat.

Little mouse approached the water and looked into it. He saw
a frightened mouse reflected there.

'Who are you?' little mouse asked the reflection. 'Are you not
afraid of being that far out into the great river?'

'No,' answered the frog, 'I am not afraid. I have been given
the gift from birth to live both above and within the river. When
winter man comes and freezes this medicine, I cannot be seen.
But all the while thunderbird flies, I am here. To visit me, one
must come when the world is green. I, my brother, am the
keeper of the water.'

'Amazing!' little mouse said at last, again fumbling for words.

'Would you like to have some medicine power?' frog asked.

'Medicine power? Me?' asked little mouse. 'Yes, yes! If it is
possible.'

'Then crouch as low as you can, and then jump as high as you
are able! You will have your medicine!' frog said.

Little mouse did as he was instructed. He crouched as low as
he could and jumped. And when he did, his eyes saw the sacred
mountains.

Little mouse could hardly believe his eyes. But there they
were! But then he fell back to Earth, and he landed in the river!

Little mouse became frightened and scrambled back to the
bank. He was wet and frightened nearly to death.

'You have tricked me,' little mouse screamed at the frog.

'Wait,' said the frog. 'You are not harmed. Do not let your
fear and anger blind you. What did you see?'

'I,' mouse stammered, 'I saw the sacred mountains!'

'And you have a new name!' frog said. 'It is Jumping Mouse.'

'Thank you. Thank you,' Jumping Mouse said, and thanked
him again. 'I want to return to my people and tell them of this
thing that has happened to me.'

'Go. Go then,' frog said. 'Return to your people. It is easy
to find them. Keep the sound of the medicine river to the back
of your head. Go opposite to the sound and you will find your
brother mice.'

Jumping Mouse returned to the world of the mice. But he
found disappointment. No one would listen to him. And
because he was wet, and had no way of explaining it because
there had been no rain, many of the other mice were afraid

of him. They believed he had been spat from the mouth of
another animal that had tried to eat him. And they all knew that
if he had not been food for the one who wanted him, then he
must also be poison for them.

Jumping Mouse lived again among his people, but he could
not forget his vision of the sacred mountains.

The memory burned in the mind and heart of Jumping
Mouse, and one day he went to the edge of the place of mice
and looked out onto the prairie. He looked up for eagles. The
sky was full of many spots, each one an eagle. But he was
determined to go to the sacred mountains. He gathered all of
his courage and ran just as fast as he could onto the prairie. His
little heart pounded with excitement and fear.

He ran until he came to a stand of sage. He was resting and
trying to catch his breath when he saw an Old Mouse. The
patch of sage Old Mouse lived in was a haven for mice. Seeds
and many things to be busy with.

'Hello,' said Old Mouse. 'Welcome.'

Jumping Mouse was amazed. Such a place and such a
mouse. 'You are truly a great mouse,' Jumping Mouse said
with all the respect that he could find. 'This is truly a wonderful place. And the eagles cannot see you here, either,' Jumping
Mouse said.

'Yes,' said Old Mouse, 'and one can see all the beings of the
prairie here: the buffalo, antelope, rabbit, and coyote. One can
see them all from here and know their names.'

'That is marvellous,' Jumping Mouse said. 'Can you also
see the river and the great mountains?'

'Yes and no,' Old Mouse said with conviction. 'I know the
great river, But I am afraid that the great mountains are only a
myth. Forget your passion to see them and stay here with me.
There is everything you want here, and it is a good place to be.'

'How can he say such a thing?' thought Jumping Mouse. 'The
medicine of the sacred mountains is nothing one can forget.'

'Thank you very much for the meal you have shared with
me, Old Mouse, and also for sharing your great home,' Jumping Mouse said. 'But I must seek the mountains.'

'You are a foolish mouse to leave, there is danger on the
prairie! Just look up there!' Old Mouse said, with even more

conviction. 'See all those spots! They are eagles, and they will catch you!'

It was hard for Jumping Mouse to leave, but he gathered his determination and ran hard again.

The ground was rough. But he arched his tail and ran with all his might. He could feel the shadows of the spots upon his back as he ran. All those spots! Finally he ran into a stand of chokecherries. Jumping Mouse could hardly believe his eyes. It was cool there and very spacious. There was water, cherries, and seeds to eat, grasses to gather for nests, holes to be explored and many, many other busy things to do. And there were a great many things to gather.

He was investigating his new domain when he heard very heavy breathing. He quickly investigated the sound and discovered its source. It was a great mound of hair with black horns. It was a great buffalo. Jumping Mouse could hardly believe the greatness of the being he saw lying there before him. He was so large that Jumping Mouse could have crawled into one of his great horns. 'Such a magnificent being,' thought Jumping Mouse, and he crept closer.

'Hello, my brother,' said the buffalo. 'Thank you for visiting me.'

'Hello Great Being,' said Jumping Mouse. 'Why are you lying here?'

'I am sick and I am dying,' the buffalo said.

'And my medicine has told me that only the eye of a mouse can heal me. But little brother, there is no such thing as a mouse.'

Jumping Mouse was shocked. 'One of my eyes!' he thought. 'One of my tiny eyes.' He scurried back into the chokecherries. But the breathing came harder and slower.

'He will die,' thought Jumping Mouse, 'if I do not give him my eye. He is too great a being to let die.'

He went back to where the buffalo lay and spoke. 'I am a mouse,' he said with a shaky voice. 'And you, my brother, are a Great Being. I cannot let you die. I have two eyes, so you may have one of them.'

The minute he said it, Jumping Mouse's eye flew out of his head and the buffalo was made whole. The buffalo jumped to his feet, shaking Jumping Mouse's whole world.

'Thank you, my little brother,' said the buffalo. 'I know of your quest for the sacred mountains and of your visit to the River. You have given me life so that I may give-away to the people. I will be your brother forever. Run under my belly and I will take you right to the foot of the sacred mountains, and you need not fear the spots. The eagles cannot see you while you run under me. All they will see will be the back of a buffalo. I am of the prairie and I will fall on you if I try to go up the mountains.'

Little mouse ran under the buffalo, secure and hidden from the spots, but with only one eye it was frightening. The buffalo's great hooves shook the whole world each time he took a step. Finally they came to a place and buffalo stopped.

'This is where I must leave you, little brother,' said the buffalo.

'Thank you very much,' said Jumping Mouse. 'But you know, it was very frightening running under you with only one eye. I was constantly in fear of your great earth-shaking hooves.'

'Your fear was for nothing,' said buffalo, 'For my way of walking is the sun dance way, and I always know where my hooves will fall. I now must return to the prairie, my brother. You can always find me there.'

Jumping Mouse immediately began to investigate his new surroundings. There were even more things here than in the other places, busier things, an abundance of seeds and other things mice like. In his investigation of these things, suddenly he ran upon a grey wolf who was sitting there doing absolutely nothing.

'Hello, brother wolf,' Jumping Mouse said.

The wolf's ears came alert and his eyes shone. 'Wolf! Wolf! Yes, that is what I am, I am a wolf!' But then his mind dimmed again and it was not long before he sat quietly again, completely without memory as to who he was. Each time Jumping Mouse reminded him who he was, he became excited, but soon would forget again.

'Such a great being,' thought Jumping Mouse, 'but he has no memory.'

Jumping Mouse went to the centre of his new place and was

quiet. He listened for a very long time to the beating of his heart. Then suddenly he made up his mind. He scurried back to where the wolf sat and he spoke.

'Brother wolf,' Jumping Mouse said.

'Wolf! Wolf,' said the wolf.

'Please brother wolf,' said Jumping Mouse, 'please listen to me. I know what will heal you. It is one of my eyes. And I want to give it to you. You are a greater being than I. I am only a mouse. Please take it.'

When Jumping Mouse stopped speaking his eye flew out of his head and the wolf was made whole.

Tears fell down the cheeks of the wolf, but his little brother could not see them, for now he was blind.

'You are a great brother,' said the wolf, 'for now I have my memory. But now you are blind. I am the guide into the sacred mountains. I will take you there. There is a great medicine lake there. The most beautiful lake in the world. All the world is reflected there. The people, the lodges of the people and all the beings of the prairies and skies.'

'Please take me there,' Jumping Mouse said. The wolf guided him through the pines to the medicine lake. Jumping Mouse drank the water from the lake. The wolf described the beauty to him.

'I must leave you here,' said wolf, 'for I must return so that I may guide others, but I will remain with you as long as you like.'

'Thank you, my brother,' said Jumping Mouse. 'But although I am frightened to be alone, I know you must go so that you may show others the way to this place.'

Jumping Mouse sat there trembling in fear. It was no use running, for he was blind, but he knew an eagle would find him here. He felt a shadow on his back and heard the sound that eagles make. He braced himself for the shock. And the eagle hit! Jumping Mouse went to sleep.

Then he woke up. The surprise of being alive was great, but now he could see!

Everything was blurry, but the colours were beautiful.

'I can see! I can see!' said Jumping Mouse, over again and again.

A blurry shape came towards Jumping Mouse. Jumping Mouse squinted hard but the shape remained a blur.

'Hello, brother,' a voice said. 'Do you want some medicine?'

'Some medicine for me?' asked Jumping Mouse. 'Yes! Yes!'

'Then crouch as low as you can,' the voice said, 'and jump as high as you can.'

Jumping Mouse did as he was instructed. He crouched as low as he could and jumped! The wind caught him and carried him higher.'

'Do not be afraid,' the voice called to him. 'Hang on to the wind and trust!'

Jumping Mouse did. He closed his eyes and hung on to the wind and it carried him higher and higher. Jumping Mouse opened his eyes and they were clear, and the higher he went the clearer they became. Jumping Mouse saw his old friend upon a lily pad on the beautiful medicine lake. It was the frog.

'You have a new name,' called the frog. 'You are Eagle!'

(The End or perhaps a new beginning)

The Four Stages of Story Medicine

Jumping Mouse is a story of change, of paradigm transformation. It tells us how our first encounter with story medicine can change our view of the world and lead us on to a journey that will eventually transform our paradigms as well as our self. The story offers a parable for the soul's path from ignorance to wisdom, from intellect to the imagination, from mouse to eagle. It is a tale that is medicinal as a whole as well as in its parts. It allows us to see deeply into the dynamics of change that are part of every transformation. One of its many gifts is to illuminate the four stages of story medicine as steps toward imaginal competence.

1. The Accidental Encounter

The first stage is the accidental encounter with story medicine. This can happen at any moment and at any time. We meet a story that speaks to us and leaves us enlivened and changed.

The very fact that a story can have this effect testifies to its medicinal properties. Our soul is met with the very imaginal boost that it needs. Like mouse, our conscious mind may know little of what it is hearing when it takes up a book or chooses a story: it is a faraway roaring that will only reveal itself in time.

2. The Use of Traditional Story

In the second stage, we actively seek stories that match our soul or the soul of others. This is the stage of the wise administration of traditional stories. Scheherazade was unrivalled master of this art with her compassionate grasp of the ailment at hand, her abundance of stories and her skill at matching them with the needs of the individual soul. We will practise this art in Part Two of this book.

Mouse enters this stage through his meeting with frog. Like Scheherazade, frog is an experienced story medic and administers the right story at the right time. With the help of powerful story medicine — the sight of the sacred mountains — frog helps mouse to see further than he has ever seen. This medicine makes mouse into Jumping Mouse. All stories matching the soul do that. They make us inwardly jump and see further than we have ever seen before. The intellect is lifted beyond its normally limiting view and is baptized with the imagination. Once we have glimpsed the sacred mountains towering at the edge of our mind we are changed. We too have a new name and know that the mountains are real.

3. Active Story-making

The third stage takes both courage and imagination. It is the stage of active story-making, where stories are created and tailored for particular soul situations. This is the art of the new Scheherazade, the creative therapist and healer of the future. It is an art that can be acquired. Story-making is indigenous to the human soul. It is familiar territory, even to one who has never been there.

Stories that are tailored for the individual soul are powerful medicine. They are effective because they are made with the recipient in mind. They are part of the imaginal conversation that links one soul with another. It is the power of imagination that makes these stories work. Seeing with the mind's eye is the active ingredient in this remedy. Through this seeing the soul gives of itself.

Jumping Mouse embarks on this stage when he heals buffalo with one of his eyes. The eye through which he has seen the sacred mountain is medicine for the beast. In other words the imagination of Jumping Mouse heals the buffalo and, through the buffalo, the land and its people — *'You have given me life so that I may give away to the people.'*

We do the same whenever we make a new story for someone. We give them the gift of our imagination, our inner seeing. This seeing is the most potent part of the remedy we prepare. But it is not only effective for the recipient. It is part of the greater ecological equation that encompasses the productions of the human mind as well as those of nature. In this equation the life of the imagination and the life of nature are close relatives. One is the artist in the world, the other in the soul. They are the same process seen from different sides. Fostering one inevitably fosters the other.

Jumping Mouse heals wolf with his second eye. His imagination awakens wolf to who wolf really is. It is only through imagination that we come to know more of who we are — and who others are. This third stage is therefore necessarily one of inner activity. The timidly-hoarding mouse becomes the generous giver of gifts. The passive recipient of story medicine becomes the active maker of it in a profound shift, which links human beings with the youngest, most vital part of themselves — the meristem of creativity, the growth point of the mind.

This is the stage of imaginal empowerment and creative activism. At this point the patient becomes the healer, the listener becomes the teller, and the reader is the new maker of tales. The soul leaves the sickbed of passivity and begins to walk towards the sacred mountain. Part Three of this book is concerned with this quest and provides a map of the territory ahead, a guide for travellers on the continent of the imagination.

4. Communion and Transformation

The fourth and final stage of story medicine is that of communion. The mouse of the intellect has come a long way and sacrificed much. Now it is time for the ultimate part of the transformation in which Jumping Mouse becomes Eagle and intellect becomes imagination. It is the stage of communion with the deeper aspect of ourselves. At this stage the telling of story becomes freed from all outer stimuli. It wings itself freely into creative action. Story becomes a product of joy rather than necessity. Free to be itself, a story born of joy frees those who hear it. Story-making has reached the stage of art. The journey of Jumping Mouse is at an end and that of Eagle is beginning, and again the frog is there to remind Jumping Mouse of who he truly is: Eagle.

Frog is the hidden story medic, the deeper knowing inside Jumping Mouse; the one who knows his names, the initiator into the realm of the imagination. The story subtly hints at this oneness with Jumping Mouse in the description of their first encounter.

> Little mouse approached the water and looked into it. He saw a frightened mouse reflected there.
>
> 'Who are you?' little mouse asked the reflection. 'Are you not afraid of being that far out into the great river?'
>
> 'No,' answered the frog, 'I am not afraid. I have been given the gift from birth to live both above and within the river. When winter man comes and freezes this medicine, I cannot be seen. But all the while thunderbird flies, I am here. To visit me, one must come when the world is green. I, my brother, am the keeper of the water.'

Mouse, ignorant about the nature of water, asks his own reflection and the frog answers in his stead. Through the frog, mouse has a conversation with his deeper self, the one that is the keeper of the water, the protector of the imagination.

There is a frog in every good story to remind us of who we are. If we listen, this frog will show us the way towards ourselves.

Each of the four stages of story medicine offers a rite of passage into creative activity. Even in the first, creative activity is present, as a receptive force. By the third stage it is fully active and in the fourth it has liberated itself from all fetters.

The first stage needs little help. It will happen by itself if we let it. The second stage is dependent on our familiarity with existing stories and our capacity to apply them in the best possible way. Part Two of this book is dedicated to this art and explores the healing potential of traditional tales.

How to raise the phoenix imagination on the wings of new story is the theme of the third part of this book.

Part 2. Traditional Tales and their Use

11. Drawing from the Universal Script

My study of story medicine in myth has confirmed my own experience with story — only the right story at the right time is true story medicine. Such stories truly speak to us. They are the rungs on the ladder the soul wishes to climb. To safely establish these rungs is the task of the next chapters.

Following the steps the imagination takes in the child and teenager I have taken my clues from childhood drawings and from the one educational model that has already developed an elaborate story culture: Waldorf Education. As far as the age-appropriate use of traditional stories is concerned, Waldorf Education provides an unprecedented standard. It may not be the only way to go about the ordering of story, but it is one that makes sense as it parallels the development of the child in the same way that childhood drawings do.

All children, irrespective of cultural and social conditions, follow the same archetypal sequence in their first attempts to draw. Whether they are born in Lapland, equatorial Africa or New York, they all start with the same kind of up and down scribbling and the grand motif of the incoming spiral. Those familiar with the development of the child can decipher this early textbook. In universal script, it describes the inner experiences taking hold in the child's body.

The incoming spiral mirrors the process of incarnation — of coming in from a greater expanse, of anchoring the suspended soul in its physical counterpart. The incoming spiral is a first ritual of childhood, the soul's dance around and into the temple of the body. The first circle shapes — returning the line into itself, or closing off the outside — coincide with the beginnings of self-consciousness. The conscious self emerges within the body like the first dot planted in the middle of the circle. At this point the child says 'I' for the first time. The brain has reached a first stage of maturation and the last separated bones in the forehead are now fused together — they too have closed the circle.

Physiology and psychology coincide and the drawings illustrate that very point. The same happens when the spine reaches maturity and towers begin to appear on the page.

The tenacity of this pattern is nowhere more apparent than in a handicapped child unable to use his hands during childhood. All the scribbles, spirals and circles remain un-drawn, but they are not lost. They are waiting to come forth, and if the handicap is lifted they will immediately do so. Thus a teenager will, without exception, go through all the missing stages in the exact sequence, although in much shorter time. Several years of drawing may be resolved into a couple of months.

This constancy points to pre-existing themes within the human soul that have a strong predisposition to surface in their own particular time. If something prevents this surfacing, they remain in waiting. By extension, this suggests an ideal sequence that the soul longs to follow, a lawfulness in its development. It may also be seen that this lawfulness echoes the steps that humanity took many ages ago.

The individual child follows these steps in its first few years, retracing the first dance as it draws on the most ancient human inheritance — the dreamtime long before any historical age.

The growing soul needs time to unfold, time to retrace, relive and re-experience the stories stored in its depths. It is the soul's birthright to linger in this dreamtime before it fully awakens. (It is during these early years, when the child is still embraced in the cocoon of dreams, that exposure to the nightmare produced by twenty-first century technology can be a traumatic experience. Violent movies and computer games can cripple the soul while it is still developing. It is the rash opening of the pupa before the butterfly has formed.)

The drawings of childhood are part of this universal story. They are the preface to all the other stories and they are written by each child. This preface is part of human nature, it happens by itself. The stories that follow in its wake, however, are already part of culture. They do not happen by themselves. They are waiting to be told.

12. The First of Tales

The first of tales is the most important tale of all.

Though we never remember it, it is the one tale we never forget. For it has become who we are. It has shaped us before we have shaped ourselves.

It is the tale of care, told by the mother in the primal language of love; it is her presence and warmth. It is a tale elaborated upon by the father, by brothers and sisters, by family and friends.

It is the long tale told before words, in the vernacular of touch, the texture of skin, the taste of milk, the cocoon of warmth. It is the story expressed through the comfort of closeness, the tone of voice, the mantle of smells; through all the changing moods that mark the seasons of family life. But most of all it is told through the mother, who sifts the coarse world through the gossamer of care.

Ideally, this is the tale that anchors us in the depth of emotion, the bond that weathers all storms. It is the tale of our first love and the blueprint for all other tales to come. It is the first of securities, the most primal of needs. It is the foundation stone on which our edifice of soul is built and it provides the matrix of our future health.

There is research which suggests that severe mental illness such as psychosis is caused by significant neglect during the first year of life. The less severe character disorders originate through abuse in the second year, and the common neuroses have their roots in the years thereafter. Human nature speaks eloquently through the high mortality rate of orphaned babies who receive the trappings of physical care but are denied emotional contact.

In this first tale, love is synonymous with life. The sustained presence of the mother or her substitute during the first years is a great gift. It helps our entry into the world and sets a precedent for our relationship to others and the world. The love received becomes the love we give. Later on the love received supports our interest in the world, our attention to others, our passion for knowledge, our ability to intimately understand, connect and fully penetrate in thought. Here, as in childhood, love makes sense.

The Language of Love

In this first tale the mother herself is the hero, for it takes courage to tell this story properly, perhaps the greatest courage of all. Nowadays, the mother is as endangered a species as the child. Without traditional family support, both mother and child suffer from the relentless persecution of love by economic pressure and the constraints of time. The natural environment of mother and child is togetherness, but they are frequently torn apart by the demands of life. The mother often has to pit herself against public opinion and pressure from family and friends.

The mother, and no one more than the single mother, is the hero of our time, the true star in the sky of childhood, the unmatched champion of love. She is the teller of the first and most important of all tales, the creation myths for those in her care.

The Mother Tongue

The expression 'mother tongue' is especially apt: language is our second mother. In the care of this mother we imbibe a whole world of nuances, attitudes and ways of seeing that are indigenous to our culture. Language structures our world. It pervades our perceptions with meaning and so shapes the way we see and how we feel about the world. Each language filters reality in unique ways.

Compare the English word *tree* with its German equivalent *baum*.

'Tree' is a straight and tall word; it emphasizes the trunk. A tree is best looked at from a distance. It can be used for ship masts and long beams. Tree is a slim, thin, longish, almost pointed word; a word that awakens, rises and moves.

'Baum' is different. It is comforting and encompassing. Baum is a steady and slow word, suggesting largeness and roundness, perhaps standing by itself on the village square with dense foliage and ample shade. People gather beneath it in the afternoon. The word 'baum' makes lovers carve love-hearts in its bark for it is an embracing word.

The Japanese equivalent is *ke* (pronounced like king without the ng). Ke immediately reminds me of a well-kept Japanese garden or a bonsai in a formal dining area. It makes me think of haiku, holding its own on a white page, and a couple of masterful brushstrokes at the edge of a Japanese painting indicating not tree, but 'ke.'

Each language suggests a way of seeing. Languages are intrinsic artworks that shape the world which in turn shapes us.

But languages do more than shape our perceptions. They teach us how to think. Languages are intelligent. As children we partake in their complex meanings long before we can master such meanings ourselves. Language contains intelligent thought like a pregnant mother contains her child. Through language, children use highly-developed, complicated and organized intelligence long before they are able to consciously produce it. Language thinks for the child and supports it on the first steps of mental independence. Language is pre-intelligence in its most artistic form.

Language as Story

Language longs to be elaborate and detailed, alive and complex. A long sentence is already on the way towards story. It carries a momentum that demands more. Thus it is good to follow sentences to the full expression they yearn towards, and take care in their formulation. It is empowering to express oneself clearly and much joy can be had from the artistic use of words. Language is the soul out loud, the open space for feelings to air themselves and the platform for meanings to meet and converse.

The language we use is a story in itself, so let us take care of it from the beginning and tell it in the right way. Like a good story, language must avoid abstraction. In childhood all abstractions are strangers. They act like alien intruders in the soul, burdening the child as with heavy lumps of undigested food. Children cannot deal with them. Intellectual content is as foreign to a child's soul as it is to a good tale.

A passage in A. A. Milne's *Winnie the Pooh* illustrates this well.

> 'I say, Owl,' said Christopher Robin, 'isn't this fun? I'm on an island!'
>
> 'The atmospheric conditions have been very unfavourable lately,' said Owl.
>
> 'The what?'
>
> 'It has been raining,' explained Owl.
>
> 'Yes,' said Christopher Robin. 'It has.'
>
> 'The flood-level has reached an unprecedented height.'
>
> 'The who?'

'There's a lot of water about,' explained Owl.

'Yes,' said Christopher Robin, 'there is.'

There's no need to be that kind of owl. Be wise rather than clever. This does not mean you have to simplify language. Your language can be as full-bodied, complex and alive as you like. The child revels in learning language from this artistic, imaginative and ensouled use.

The Childhood of Language

Children with brothers and sisters are lucky. Siblings are reliable company. They are our first community and the perfect opportunity to learn the human trade of give and take, closeness and distance. The mothering tongue also provides us with siblings — the hums and songs, play-languages and nursery rhymes that populate our early years, as playful as any brother or sister.

The hum comes first. Born at the same time as we are, she is our delicate twin-sister (the ruffian nursery rhyme is the older brother). The hum continues the music of the womb. It is the softest of all songs, the swaddling clothes woven from the mother's voice. It envelops the child like a cocoon, soothing its entrance into the world of sound. The hum is the first music, a primal song in which mother and nature still coincide. Like a slow, warm, steady cradle it calms the baby into contentment.

Hums belong to the first of tales, the tale of care. They weave babe and mother into one undivided whole and then flow into the lullaby. The lullaby is more of the world, and soon grows into little ditties and songs.

During the early years songs are best sung by the mother or father or other members of the household, for their main purpose is the assurance of human presence.

Not so long ago, singing had a continuous presence in human life. It was part of almost every human activity. Mothers hummed and sang. Men and women worked to the rhythm of ploughing, sowing and harvest songs; scything songs and milking songs. Each trade and guild had its songs. Songs were woven into the stitches of the cobbler and the weaving of women; the carvings of woodcutters and the whip of horsemen. There were songs for the morning and for the evening, for summer and autumn, winter and spring. Every festival fostered song and every church and temple, synagogue and mosque was a place for music.

In childhood, hums and songs are soon followed by finger plays and rhyming games. Rhymes like 'This little piggy went to market' are learned on the mother's lap. Being together turns into doing together, and language is joined by touch and tickle. Movement and language coincide and in turn stimulate the brain.

Nursery rhymes have already jumped from the mother's lap. They are more adventurous siblings than finger plays. They don't need to be learned, they are already known. Children meet them like old possessions or long-lost friends. They are playmates made of ianguage. Through them an ancient layer of language echoes in modern form. They are a version of the old magical invocation. Even today they act like spells, charming us forever. They seize us the moment we hear them and they never release us. When we have long forgotten other verse we still know them by heart.

Nursery rhymes are little rituals chanted in groups, compelling us to move and dance and step and clap. Rhythm, repetition and rhyme prevail over meaning. And yet they are also miniature tales, stories provided by language itself. Each is an embryonic myth, a long-lost knowledge encoded in pictures. They are our first poetic experience, our opportunity to dance with the genius of English from little stories into the ballroom of larger tales. These rhymes belong to story medicine. They are primal medicine, like good food and joy. Nursery rhymes are indeed the nursery of all other tales; they are the stories we start with.

13. The Body of Story

Leaving the nursery of rhymes it is time to sow our first stories. The next couple of chapters are a kind of planting calendar that will help you to plant the right story at the right time. Take my suggestions as a stimulus only. Stories naturally resist confinement; a proper tale changes all the time. It is always unruly, too alive to be tamed; a chameleon whose natural environment is the context in which it is told.

The listener is part of this context for it is only in the listener's imagination that stories come truly alive. It is the listener who gives them final shape and makes them into what they are. Much, therefore, depends on the child who hears them. For this reason I will suggest an ideal time for a story to be told, although obviously there may be children of four who are ready for a six year old's tale.

The reception of story depends also on the relationship of the child to the adult. Familiarity and trust in the storyteller are prerequisites for the medicinal action of story. And of course, much also depends on the teller, on his or her relationship to the story and how it is told.

A story needs to be loved and respected by the narrator to fully unfold in a child's soul. It is best told in a quiet space, with ample time on either side, and in a calm and natural voice. Stories for a young child need no added drama. Leave that to the imagination of the child — she will know what to do. When you over-emphasize words or passages, you are imposing your interpretation on the child. You force her to give importance to what is important to you. This does not leave her free to receive the story unmediated and nor does it respect the story for what it is — now it comes with your agenda attached.

When a story is read or told according to these principles, the listener is free to decode it in her own way. This is particularly important when children of different ages are assembled. It will not always do to adjust the story to the youngest; in fact I recommend you consciously address the story to the oldest child. In this way younger siblings will take only what they are prepared for. Their imagination may pick at the pebbles that Hansel has left on the trail while the older child is impatiently waiting for Gretel to push the witch into the oven.

Sweet Porridge (age three)

The tales that follow songs and nursery rhymes need to be simple at first. At the age of three the child is ready to digest a story like Sweet Porridge.

> There was a poor but good little girl who lived alone with her mother, and they no longer had anything to eat. So the child went into the forest, and there an aged woman met her who was aware of her sorrow, and presented her with a little pot, which when she said, 'Cook, little pot, cook,' would cook good, sweet porridge, and when she said, 'Stop, little pot,' it ceased to cook. The girl took the pot home to her mother, and now they were freed from their poverty and hunger, and ate sweet porridge as often as they chose.
>
> Once when the girl had gone out, her mother said, 'Cook, little pot, cook.' And it did cook and she ate till she was satisfied, and then she wanted the pot to stop cooking, but did not know the word. So it went on cooking and the porridge rose over the edge, and still it cooked on until the kitchen and whole house were full, and then the next house, and then the whole street, just as if it wanted to satisfy the hunger of the whole world, and there was the greatest distress, but no one knew how to stop it. At last when only one single house remained, the child came home and just said, 'Stop, little pot,' and it stopped and gave up cooking, and whosoever wished to return to the town had to eat his way back.

Sweet Porridge celebrates the competence of the small child. Rightly understood, this story is an initiation into the power of language, a power that the child is acquiring at this stage.

To the very young child, food is a first form of communication, a kind of primal language learned at the mother's breast. Many of the child's first utterances are related to hunger and thirst. In time the child learns that words have the power to procure food as well as to make it disappear.

Through her first experiences she learns that the spoken word is a power greater than food; greater than hunger and thirst, needs and wants. She learns that language resides above this realm and has command of it. And so does the one who uses it. She who speaks overcomes the compulsion of needs by the power of the 'right word' and so establishes the sovereignty of being human over the mute world of wants. All this and more is contained in Sweet Porridge. It's a substantial dish at the age of three and even before. Like the pot in the story it will nourish both you and your child. And you need not worry when to stop this kind of meal. The child will know the word.

Other stories you can add to your menu for the three to four year old are: *Goldilocks and the Three Bears, The Farmer who went to Plough* and *The Gingerbread Man.*

The Three Billy Goats Gruff (age four)

Stories for a four year old can include *The Elves and the Shoemaker* and the much loved Norwegian folktale of *The Three Billy Goats Gruff. The Three Billy Goats Gruff* is a favourite of children at this age and beyond. I have heard of a boy who wanted this story every day until he was twelve and still asked for it occasionally years after that (which just goes to show that *The Three Billy Goats Gruff* is a story useful for any stage of life). And in case it is useful for you right now, I include it here.

> Once on a time there were three billy goats, who were to go up to the hillside to make themselves fat, and the name of all three was 'Gruff.'
>
> On the way up was a bridge over a stream they had to cross; and under the bridge lived a great ugly Troll, with eyes as big as saucers, and a nose as long as a poker.
>
> So first of all came the youngest billy goat Gruff to cross the bridge.
>
> 'Trip, trap! trip, trap!' went the bridge.
>
> 'WHO'S THAT tripping over my bridge?' roared the Troll.
>
> 'Oh, it is only I, the tiniest billy goat Gruff; and I'm going up to the hillside to make myself fat,' said the billy goat, with such a small voice.
>
> 'Now, I'm coming to gobble you up,' said the Troll.
>
> 'Oh, no! pray don't take me. I'm too little,' said the billy goat; 'wait a bit till the second billy goat Gruff comes, he's much bigger.'
>
> 'Well, be off with you,' said the Troll.

A little while after came the second billy goat Gruff to cross the bridge.

'TRIP, TRAP! TRIP, TRAP! TRIP, TRAP!' went the bridge.

'WHO'S THAT tripping over my bridge?' roared the Troll.

'Oh, it's the second billy goat Gruff, and I'm going up to the hillside to make myself fat,' said the billy goat, who hadn't such a small voice.

'Now I'm coming to gobble you up,' said the Troll.

'Oh, no! don't take me, wait a little till the big billy goat Gruff comes, he's much bigger.'

'Very well! be off with you,' said the Troll.

But just then up came the big billy goat Gruff.

'TRIP, TRAP! TRIP, TRAP! TRIP, TRAP!' went the bridge, for the big billy goat was so heavy that the bridge creaked and groaned under him.

'WHO'S THAT tramping over my bridge?' roared the Troll.

'IT'S I! THE BIG BILLY GOAT GRUFF,' said the billy goat, who had an ugly hoarse voice of his own.

'Now I'm coming to gobble you up,' roared the Troll.

'Well, come along! I've got two spears,

And I'll poke your eyeballs out at your ears;

I've got besides two curling-stones,

And I'll crush you to bits, body and bones.'

That was what the big billy goat said; and so he flew at the Troll, and poked his eyes out with his horns, and crushed him to bits, body and bones, and tossed him out into the stream, and after that he went up to the hillside. There the billy goats got so fat they were scarce able to walk home again; and if the fat hasn't fallen off them, why, they're still fat; and so —

Snip, snap, snout

This tale's told out.

The reason young children like this story and why the boy liked it for so long and why you might like it even now is that it addresses the cycles of growth. It is about growing up, maturation and mastery. Growing up is a lifelong business. It is never finished; there is always more of it ahead of us. At heart we always remain a child who is humble enough to know our true size in the larger affair of being human.

The child is in this state by necessity — acutely aware of her limitations and dependencies. Almost everything is yet to be learned, acquired, achieved. Mastery is a long way off. To begin with, even the tying of shoe-laces is an arcane art, and reading and writing a miraculous accomplish-ment. Every machine is a riddle, every adult a numinous being.

Between now and the future, between the child and the adult, between helplessness and competence, there lies a bridge: the bridge of time. Beneath it lurks the challenge, the resistance, the troll. But the bridge has to be crossed to get from here to there. To do this safely requires wit, humility and above all knowledge of the right time — and the patience to wait for it. The three billy goats Gruff have this patience. The first two know that their time has not yet come. They know they have to wait. But they also know that the time will come for the third billy goat Gruff — the one who *can* master the troll.

Children need to know this. They need to know that their time will come too. That it is worthwhile to wait and trust in the future. That the one who waits in patience for the right moment to arrive will meet every challenge. This is what the three billy goats Gruff teach. They are mas-ters of timing. Just like a good storyteller they know when to do what.

Heroes at Five, Six, Seven

From the age of five, stories like *The Frog Prince, Mother Holle, The Bremen Town Musicians* and *Sleeping Beauty* are appropriate (they can all be found on our website: *www.sofia.net.au*). This is not to say that these stories ought not to be told *before* the age of five. But the full impact of the heroic journey will only be fully appreciated after the child has established an inner centre of initiative — in other words, when she has found the hero within. Only then can she understand the nature of a quest and all it contains: the personal challenge, the overcoming of obstacles and the meeting with evil.

The safest way to encounter evil is on the parent's lap and in the form of story. A tale like *Mother Holle* offers a highly integrated opportunity to meet evil where it is most readily to be found: in one's own soul. *Mother Holle* masterfully addresses the higher and lower aspects of the psyche through the two girls, one of whom is industrious and fair while the other is ugly and lazy. The child will instinctively feel that both girls are one, that every human being has a golden side and a pitch-black side. The story hints at this in the way the two girls have exactly the same experiences.

In stories appropriate for the five to six year old, evil is kept at bay. It is part of the story, but not central to it. The thirteenth wise woman who curses the Sleeping Beauty and causes her to sleep for a hundred years is still a marginal character.

With stories appropriate to the six or seven year old, the confrontation with evil moves to centre stage. The wolf in *Little Red Riding Hood* is a major player. Even so, children understand that the Wolf is a figure in soul space, not in reality. They know that the drama is imaginative rather than literal, that there is no bloodshed when the wolf devours the grandmother and no need to wipe the floor after he has gobbled up the child. Nor does the hunter need anaesthetic to rescue Red Riding Hood and her grandmother from the wolf's belly. They are still whole inside the wolf.

In contrast to many adults, children understand metaphoric reality. They know how to take stories seriously in their own right and they live wholeheartedly in the pictures they provide. That is why the household tale is such an indispensable tool in preparing children for the world. Each fairytale provides the utmost education in a minimal form. The learning is effortless. Insights are served on the golden plate of the imagination and morality is conveyed without being preached.

The best way to ascertain whether your child is ready to meet the more complex fairytales is by means of a test or trial. Once this test is passed the child will have found her own centre of initiative, the hero within. The emergence of this hero is the sure sign that the child is able to deal with the challenges that the more adventurous fairytales provide. The test I am talking about is the trial of boredom.

The Trial of Boredom (age five)

Boredom is a modern epidemic. It is persuasive and highly infectious. Boredom has two faces: one that is bored not knowing what to do and one that is bored whatever it does. The faces are identical twins; it is hard to tell which is which.

Such patterns often have their origin in childhood. The problem of boredom comes in many guises and it begins to court us seriously at the age of five. If it is not dealt with then, it may weave itself into the fabric of our life. It either finds a hidden niche to wait or it is kept unashamedly as a favourite pet. Boredom's most outstanding feature is its insatiability:

the more it is fed the more it writhes in contortions of hunger. It is unfailingly opportunistic and is always ready to pounce on our time.

But do not despair. There is a remedy in the form of a well-known story that will effect an immediate cure as well as a long-term preventative. Once learned it can be used with great effect. You may know a variation of this story already, at least in part. It is the tale of Dragon Fare and comes in two parts.

Part One: Siege of the Old City

Jack:	Mum?
Mum:	Yes, my darling?
Jack:	I don't know what to do.
Mum:	Why don't you go outside and play in the sandpit?
Jack:	I don't want to play in the sandpit. It's boring.
	(Pause)
Jack:	Mum!
Mum:	Yes.
Jack:	Could you phone Tim again. They might be back by now …
Mum:	I've phoned twice already. They're not home. And Dan is in Albany with his dad. And Ruben is sick.
Jack:	Can I watch TV? There's …

This story is a kind of domestic *Iliad*. The old city (Mum) is under siege. A dread army (Jack) has surrounded her, battering the gates, climbing the walls, storming the ramparts. The attackers work with cunning and force. They are determined to fight to the bitter end.

The defenders are exhausted. Their forces are tied up in domestic tasks. Friends and allies are engaged elsewhere (away for the weekend, struck by sickness). All calls for help have remained unanswered. The situation is dire. In this moment of crisis the invincible commander in chief (Mum) saves the city and herself through sheer presence of mind.

Mum: I'm so glad you have some time on your hands. I need a bit of help. You can start with drying up the dishes …

There are as many variations to this part of the story as there are chores in a household. Sometimes the story ends here. At other times it has only just begun.

Part Two: In the Dragon's Lair

The war against the Old City has been raging for a while. Attracted by the noise, the fire and the smoke, the dragon has arrived. It is suddenly there.

Jack is only dimly aware of the dragon's arrival, but Mum can clearly see it when Jack slinks angrily away from the dishes, darkly muttering, smoking with fury, stamping with open rage, slamming doors and spitting fire.

The dragon sticks to Jack like a shadow, wherever he goes: to his bedroom, into the back yard, to the sandpit. The dragon's lair is everywhere and there is no escape. The beast of frustration bars his way at every gate. Its gaze is hypnotic. Its power is real.

But in the midst of the black cave of anger a spark suddenly disperses the darkness. Jack has a new idea and it cuts like a lance through the thick scales of the dragon, right into the belly of its boredom, and with one stroke of childhood genius his world is rid of despair.

With one last puff of smoke the dragon falls, rolls over and reveals, right there, hidden till that moment beneath its foul apathetic body, a treasure hoard of silver coins and golden opportunity, gems of new ideas, scrolls of untried plans and treasure maps, flying carpets ready to take off and lamps complete with genies willing to transform sandpits into castles and sparse trees into the dense woods of adventures.

The Birth of the Hero

The trial of boredom begins when nothing entertains us any more. It ends when we begin to entertain ourselves. In the gap in between is the birthplace of the hero.

Outwardly nothing has changed, but a battle has been won. A hero has emerged. An explorer has found himself in the dragon's lair, an inventor has discovered himself in the smoky cavern of the beast and a storyteller is born in the womb of his own tale.

Boredom and creativity are closely related. The same force is manifest in each. Boredom becomes creativity by dint of inner effort. Creativity turns into boredom through lack of effort.

The strength called on by the parent sparks a similar strength in the child. The battle cannot be avoided. It has to be won again and again against the paralysis of giving in to the immediate want, the easy distraction. If it is not fought then relief is short-lived and the consequences life-long. The dragon drags on. Its hunger, it bears saying again, is insatiable. The more it is fed the more it will grow in power and sophistication. The only way to overcome this dragon is for the hero to meet it and transform it.

If the trial is mastered, initiative takes the place of apathy and imagination replaces boredom. The child that has hitherto been sparked only by the dazzle of outer events and the offer of toys is now increasingly motivated from within. New ideas begin to surface and plans are made independent of outer circumstance, which are now arranged by the child to suit his intentions rather than the reverse. In other words, the hero has begun to emerge.

A true hero needs a tale as much as a tale needs a hero. The child's imagination is now ready for a new step. Like the fairytale, it is ready to imaginatively face evil in whatever form evil appears. Most likely it will first come in some sort of disguise, perhaps as a gingerbread house.

Hansel and Gretel (age six or seven)

The depth and complexity with which the household tale addresses the problem of evil is marvellously transparent in the story of *Hansel and Gretel*, included it here for those who have not met it in its entirety.

> Hard by a great forest dwelt a poor woodcutter with his wife and his two children. The boy was called Hansel and the girl Gretel. He had little to bite and to break, and when great dearth fell on the land, he could no longer procure even daily bread. Now when he thought over this by night in his bed, and tossed about in his anxiety, he groaned and said to his wife: 'What is to become of us? How are we to feed our poor children, when we no longer have anything even for ourselves?'
>
> 'I'll tell you what, husband,' answered the woman, 'early tomorrow morning we will take the children out into the forest to where it is thickest; there we will light a fire for them, and give each of them one more piece of bread, and then we will

go to our work and leave them alone. They will not find the way home again, and we shall be rid of them.'

'No, wife,' said the man, 'I will not do that; how can I bear to leave my children alone in the forest — the wild animals would soon come and tear them to pieces.'

'O, you fool!' said she, 'then we must all four die of hunger, you may as well plane the planks for our coffins,' and she left him no peace until he consented. 'But I feel very sorry for the poor children, all the same,' said the man.

The two children had also not been able to sleep for hunger, and had heard what their stepmother had said to their father. Gretel wept bitter tears, and said to Hansel: 'Now all is over with us.'

'Be quiet, Gretel,' said Hansel, 'do not distress yourself, I will soon find a way to help us.' And when the old folks had fallen asleep, he got up, put on his little coat, opened the door below, and crept outside. The moon shone brightly, and the white pebbles which lay in front of the house glittered like silver pennies. Hansel stooped and stuffed the little pocket of his coat with as many as he could fit. Then he went back and said to Gretel: 'Be comforted, little sister, and sleep in peace, God will not forsake us,' and he lay down again in his bed.

When day dawned, but before the sun had risen, the woman came and awoke the two children, saying: 'Get up, you sluggards! We are going into the forest to fetch wood.' She gave each a little piece of bread, and said: 'There is something for your dinner, but do not eat it up before then, for you will get nothing else.' Gretel took the bread under her apron, as Hansel had the pebbles in his pocket. Then they all set out together on the way to the forest. When they had walked a short time, Hansel stopped and peeped back at the house, and did so again and again. His father said: 'Hansel, what are you looking at there and lagging behind for? Pay attention, and do not forget how to use your legs.'

'Ah, father,' said Hansel, 'I am looking at my little white cat, which is sitting up on the roof, and wants to say goodbye to me.' The wife said: 'Fool, that is not your little cat, that is the morning sun which is shining on the chimneys.' Hansel, however, had not been looking back at the cat, but had been constantly throwing one of the white pebble-stones out of his pocket onto the road.

When they had reached the middle of the forest, the father said: 'Now, children, pile up some wood, and I will light a fire that you may not be cold.' Hansel and Gretel gathered brushwood together, as high as a little hill. The brushwood was lighted, and when the flames were burning very high, the woman said: 'Now, children, lay yourselves down by the fire and rest, we will go into the forest and cut some wood. When we have done, we will come back and fetch you away.'

Hansel and Gretel sat by the fire, and when noon came, each ate a little piece of bread, and as they heard the strokes of the wood-axe they believed that their father was near. It was not the axe, however, but a branch which he had fastened to a withered tree which the wind was blowing backwards and forwards. And as they had been sitting such a long time, their eyes closed with fatigue, and they fell fast asleep. When at last they awoke, it was already dark night. Gretel began to cry and said: 'How are we to get out of the forest now?' But Hansel comforted her and said: 'Just wait a little, until the moon has risen, and then we will soon find the way.' And when the full moon had risen, Hansel took his little sister by the hand, and followed the pebbles which shone like newly-coined silver pieces, and showed them the way.

They walked the whole night long, and by break of day came once more to their father's house. They knocked at the door, and when the woman opened it and saw that it was Hansel and Gretel, she said: 'You naughty children, why have you slept so long in the forest — we thought you were never coming back at all!' The father, however, rejoiced, for it had cut him to the heart to leave them behind alone.

Not long afterwards, there was once more great dearth throughout the land, and the children heard their mother saying at night to their father: 'Everything is eaten again, we have one half loaf left, and that is the end. The children must go, we will take them farther into the wood, so that they will not find their way out again; there is no other means of saving ourselves!' The man's heart was heavy, and he said: 'It would be better to share the last mouthful with the children.' The woman, however, would listen to nothing that he had to say, but scolded and reproached him. He who says A must say B, likewise, and as he had yielded the first time, he had to do so a second time also.

The children, however, were also awake and had heard the conversation. When the old folks were asleep, Hansel again got up to go out and pick up pebbles as he had done before, but the woman had locked the door, and he could not get out. Nevertheless he comforted his little sister, and said: 'Do not cry, Gretel, go to sleep quietly, the good God will help us.'

Early in the morning came the woman, and took the children out of their beds. Their piece of bread was given to them, but it was still smaller than the time before. On the way into the forest Hansel crumbled his in his pocket, and often stood still and threw a morsel on the ground. 'Hansel, why do you stop and look round,' said the father, 'go on.'

'I am looking back at my little pigeon which is sitting on the roof, and wants to say good-bye to me,' answered Hansel. 'Fool!' said the woman, 'that is not your little pigeon, that is the morning sun shining on the chimney.' Hansel, however, little by little, threw all the crumbs on the path.

The woman led the children still deeper into the forest, where they had never in their lives been before. Then a great fire was again made, and the mother said: 'Just sit there, you children, and when you are tired you may sleep a little; we are going into the forest to cut wood, and in the evening when we are done, we will come and fetch you away.' When it was noon, Gretel shared her piece of bread with Hansel, who had scattered his by the way. Then they fell asleep and evening passed, but no one came to the poor children. They did not awake until it was dark night, and Hansel comforted his little sister and said: 'Just wait, Gretel, until the moon rises, and then we shall see the crumbs of bread which I have strewn about, they will show us our way home again.'

When the moon came they set out, but they found no crumbs, for the many birds which fly about in the woods and fields had picked them all up. Hansel said to Gretel: 'We shall soon find the way,' but they did not find it. They walked the whole night and all the next day too, from morning till

evening, but they did not get out of the forest, and were very
hungry, for they had nothing to eat but two or three berries,
which grew on the ground. And as they were so weary that
their legs would carry them no longer, they lay down beneath a
tree and fell asleep.

It was now three mornings since they had left their father's
house. They began to walk again, but they always came deeper
into the forest, and if help did not come soon, they must die of
hunger and weariness. When it was midday, they saw a beautiful snow-white bird sitting on a bough, which sang so delight-
fully that they stood still and listened to it. And when its song
was over, it spread its wings and flew away before them, and
they followed it until they reached a little house, on the roof of
which it alighted; and when they approached the little house
they saw that it was made of gingerbread and covered with
cakes, but that the windows were of clear sugar. 'We will set to
work on that,' said Hansel, 'and have a good meal. I will eat a
bit of the roof, and you Gretel, can eat some of the window, it
will be sweet.' Hansel reached up above, and broke off a little
of the roof to try how it tasted, and Gretel leaned against the
window and nibbled at the panes. Then a soft voice cried from
the parlour:

'Nibble, nibble, gnaw,

'Who is nibbling at my little house?'

The children answered:

'The wind, the wind,

'The heaven-born wind,' and went on eating without dis-
turbing themselves.

Hansel, who liked the taste of the roof, tore down a great
piece of it, and Gretel pushed out the whole of one round win-
dow-pane, sat down, and enjoyed herself with it. Suddenly the
door opened, and a woman as old as the hills, who supported
herself on crutches, came creeping out. Hansel and Gretel
were so terribly frightened that they let fall what they had in
their hands. The old woman, however, nodded her head, and
said: 'Oh, you dear children, who has brought you here? Do
come in, and stay with me. No harm shall happen to you.' She
took them both by the hand, and led them into her little house.
Then good food was set before them, milk and pancakes, with

sugar, apples, and nuts. Afterwards two pretty little beds were covered with clean white linen, and Hansel and Gretel lay down in them, and thought they were in heaven.

The old woman had only pretended to be so kind, however; she was in reality a wicked witch, who lay in wait for children, and had only built the little house of gingerbread in order to entice them there. When a child fell into her power, she killed it, cooked and ate it, and that was a feast day with her. Witches have red eyes, and cannot see far, but they have a keen scent like the beasts, and are aware when human beings draw near. When Hansel and Gretel had come into her neighbourhood, she had laughed with malice, and said mockingly: 'I have them, they shall not escape me again!'

Early in the morning before the children were awake, she was already up, and when she saw them sleeping and looking so pretty, with their plump and rosy cheeks, she muttered to herself: 'That will be a dainty mouthful.' Then she seized Hansel with her shrivelled hand, carried him into a little stable, and locked him behind a grated door. Scream as he might, it would not help. Then she went to Gretel, shook her till she awoke, and cried: 'Get up, lazy thing, fetch some water, and cook something good for your brother, he is in the stable outside, and is to be made fat. When he is fat, I will eat him.' Gretel began to weep bitterly, but it was in vain, for she was forced to do what the wicked witch commanded.

And now the best food was cooked for poor Hansel, but Gretel got nothing but crab-shells. Every morning the woman crept to the little stable, and cried: 'Hansel, stretch out your finger that I may feel if you will soon be fat.' Hansel, however, stretched out a little bone to her, and the old woman, who had dim eyes, could not see it, and thought it was Hansel's finger, and was astonished that there was no way of fattening him. When four weeks had gone by, and Hansel still remained thin, she was seized with impatience and would not wait any longer. 'Now, then, Gretel,' she cried to the girl, 'stir yourself, and bring some water. Let Hansel be fat or lean, tomorrow I will kill him and cook him.' Ah, how the poor little sister did lament when she had to fetch the water, and how her tears did flow down her cheeks! 'Dear God, do help us,' she cried. 'If the wild beasts in the forest had but devoured us, we should at any rate have died together.'

'Just keep your noise to yourself,' said the old woman, 'it won't help you at all.' Early in the morning, Gretel had to go out and hang up the cauldron with the water and light the fire. 'We will bake first,' said the old woman, 'I have already heated the oven, and kneaded the dough.' She pushed poor Gretel out to the oven, from which flames of fire were already darting. 'Creep in,' said the witch, 'and see if it is properly heated, so that we can put the bread in.' For once Gretel was inside, she intended to shut the oven and let her bake in it, and then she would eat her, too. But Gretel saw what she had in mind, and said: 'I do not know how I am to do it; how do I get in?'

'Silly goose,' said the old woman. 'The door is big enough; just look, I can get in myself!' and she crept up and thrust her head into the oven. Then Gretel gave her a push that drove her far into it, and shut the iron door, and fastened the bolt. Oh then she began to howl quite horribly, but Gretel ran away, and the godless witch was miserably burnt to death.

Gretel ran like lightning to Hansel, opened his little stable, and cried: 'Hansel, we are saved! The old witch is dead!' Then Hansel sprang like a bird from its cage when the door is opened. How they did rejoice and embrace each other, and dance about and kiss each other! And as they had no longer any need to fear her, they went into the witch's house, and in every corner there stood chests full of pearls and jewels. 'These are far better than pebbles!' said Hansel, and thrust into his pockets whatever could be fit in, and Gretel said: 'I, too, will take something home with me,' and filled her pinafore full. 'But now we must be off,' said Hansel, 'that we may get out of the witch's forest.'

When they had walked for two hours, they came to a great stretch of water. 'We cannot cross,' said Hansel, 'I see no foot-plank, and no bridge.'

'And there is no ferry,' answered Gretel, 'but a white duck is swimming there; if I ask her, she will help us over.' Then she cried:

'Little duck, little duck, dost thou see,
Hansel and Gretel are waiting for thee?

There's never a plank, or bridge in sight,
Take us across on thy back so white.'

The duck came to them, and Hansel seated himself on its back, and told his sister to sit by him. 'No,' replied Gretel, 'that will be too heavy for the little duck; she shall take us across, one after the other.' The good little duck did so, and when they were safely across and had walked for a short time, the forest seemed to be more and more familiar to them, and at length they saw from afar their father's house. Then they began to run, rushed into the parlour, and threw themselves round their father's neck. The man had not known one happy hour since he had left the children in the forest; the woman, however, was dead. Gretel emptied her pinafore until pearls and precious stones ran about the room, and Hansel threw one handful after another out of his pocket to add to them. Then all anxiety was at an end, and they lived together in perfect happiness.

Hansel and Gretel is a tale for any child between the age of six and one hundred and six. It is appropriate at almost any time in life for it addresses important issues involved in any process of change and transformation.

As in *Sweet Porridge* and *The Three Billy Goats Gruff,* food plays a central part. Hansel and Gretel are abandoned for the lack of food, when the 'great dearth fell upon the land.' But there is more to the story than the age-old tale of need tied to the heel of those who leave the golden age of home.

First of all there are two heroes: a brother and a sister. The story strikes a rare balance in fairytale between the masculine and feminine elements — Hansel is more active in the beginning of the adventure, Gretel at the end. It is her mixture of wit and courage that saves them both.

The story of *Hansel and Gretel* contains many layers of meaning and poetic detail. I have always loved the scene when Hansel looks back at the house and with his childhood imagination sees the white cat on the roof where his stepmother sees only the chimney lit by the morning sun. And I am always intrigued by the little bird of guidance that leads them to the gingerbread hut and the little duck that helps them return home.

The Sweet House of Addiction

What makes *Hansel and Gretel* so pertinent for our times is the way it addresses the topic of attachment and addiction in relation to the process of 'leaving home.' The parting from home occupies almost half of the tale. Parting is never easy and takes time. In the story it has to be undertaken twice: the first time, the children return. The second time they remain lost.

The world is always a place of lack and always contains a stepmother who will make us leave, wherever we are. Most of our life is about leaving home. We leave home when we are born, when our mother weans us, when we are taken to childcare. We leave the familiarity of kindergarten for school, the comfort of childhood for puberty, our peer group at high school for new experiences in the world at large. We leave home for our first flat, and we leave it when we enter a relationship or terminate a marriage, change jobs or move to another country. After forty we leave the comfortable home of our youthful looks and unquestioned health and some twenty years later we leave the home of professional life. The last home we leave is the first we inhabit: our body.

As in the story, parting is never easy and we want to return. When that is impossible, we feel lost. All kinds of insecurities lurk beyond the fence of the familiar. Left alone and to our own devices we wander in the 'dark wood'. Like Hansel and Gretel we are desperate and in need. And like them we will find the gingerbread house. There are many such houses in life. And they always answer to our direst need, our lack. If we are hungry it will be bread and cake; if we are alone it will be a relationship; if we are ambitious, it will be money or fame. And the new job or partner or house or opportunity will make us feel as if we are in heaven. But the sweeter the house, the more sour it is likely to turn. At the extremities of this story we find ourselves locked into the cage of addiction. All Hansels end up behind bars and all Gretels are made handmaids to terrible schemes.

Life is a long series of leave-takings, feeling lost and falling prey to sweet houses. But it is equally a series of liberations. Every sweet house turned sour is an opportunity. It is the challenge that spurs our return to ourselves — laden with the treasure of experience.

To break the pattern of addiction is not easy. It takes courage and insight. Through her presence of mind Gretel sees through the schemes of their captor and with courage she does to the witch as the witch had intended to do with her. The witch — that is the addiction — burns in the fire of her own making, 'howling quite horribly.' This is what addictions do when we try to stop them. They burn in their own fire and so consume themselves.

We have all heard the cry of craving gnawing on its own bone. We know it in many variations: we cry when we are born, the baby howls when it is deprived of its breast and teenagers sob when a relationship ends. We know the quiet howl of stopping smoking, the extended howl of a traumatic divorce and the head-banging howl of addicts going cold turkey.

But after the howling comes the satisfaction of having overcome the terror: Hansel's liberation. Then there is the joy of freedom, of finding the treasures, and of the final return when the attachment is overcome, the addiction conquered. The treasures are the wisdom we gain through facing the challenge. It is what we bring home. The pain endured makes us compassionate. We are no longer the same. Nor are Hansel and Gretel: when a duck offers to take them over a great stretch of water, Gretel insists on going one by one, so as not to overburden the bird.

Every challenge we master does the same for us. It makes us more mature and leaves us with treasure to share.

In *Hansel and Gretel* this theme is not restricted to individual lives. It applies to all levels of human existence. It may be applied to a marriage, to the life of a corporation, to the destiny of a people or a culture. At its highest level the story provides a metaphor for the life of humanity.

The witch plays a prominent part in this tale. Many interpretations see the evil witch figure as a patriarchal device. I take a different view. To me the household tales bear the mark of the imagination, the feminine side of creativity. They are primarily women's lore. The Brothers Grimm merely collected these stories from the women who held them. The witch of the folktale is an archetype of interior dimension that has little to do with the millions of women persecuted and burned at the stake by bigoted churchmen.

The witch in the household tales is the imagination's way of dealing with the feminine shadow in both women and men. It is an original creation of female spirituality and ought to be honoured as such.

14. Legends and Saints

Legend and Fable (seven and eight)

Legends have left the pure air of the imagination on which the fairytale thrives and have descended to earth: placed in time and space they are linked to memorable events. Often they are history dressed in story. Their protagonists may be the saints who conquered themselves or the heroes who conquered others.

While traditional household tales are the offspring of the imagination, legends are products of the intellect. This links them to their older cousin, the fable, also fathered by the intellect. The fable uses the metaphor to illustrate moral concepts and ideas. The moral it contains is often given as a homily at the end. In the fable of the fox and the grapes, the moral is: 'It is easy to despise what you cannot get.'

This is typical of the intellect, which likes to obscure its schemes. For in truth the moral that stands at the end stood already at the inception of the tale: the purpose of the fable was to illustrate this particular moral, by means of imagination that is opportunistically added. The authentic use of imagination is as far out of reach of the moralising intellect as the grapes are for the fox. And just like the fox, the fable manages to obscure its disappointment with a cunning scheme.

But in spite of this, and maybe even because of it, fables and the legends of the saints offer themselves as a bridge between the world of imagination and the world of intellect. For the intellect cracks the world in two and opens up an abyss that the soul must cross. The child of seven or eight crosses this bridge into a new reality and the fables and legends help secure this transition. They are like the railings that give the child a secure hold.

Fable and legend separate the integrated world of the fairytale into two distinct parts. Where a household tale integrates the polarity between the moral dimensions of good and evil and resolves them in the process of transformation, fable and legend deal with them separately.

Aesop's Fables deal with the unsavoury aspects of the human soul. This is appropriate to the eight year old child. Children at this age become 'clever' and the cleverly devised fable meets them on their own ground. It works like a homeopathic: clothed in the form of fable, the intellect treats the very illness it causes. The intellect is linked to the rise in egoism and the fable holds a mirror to its baser inclinations.

The saint legends do the same for the higher self. While the fable tends to portray vices in the form of animals, the legends depict virtues in the lives of saints and heroes. Between them, legend and fable provide a balanced picture of the human soul. The child needs such a picture to orient herself in the world she is slowly awakening to. Part of this world is her own soul-life and her first conscious experience of light and dark, moral and virtue. When she hears a well-rendered fable like the Wolf and the Stork she will become more aware of what she has already experienced in herself.

> Wolves have a name for appetite
> And one upon a festive night
> Bolted his meal so greedily
> They say, he nearly breathed his last
> Far down his throat a bone stuck fast
> He could not even raise a cry.
> By lucky chance a stork flew by
> And saw him signalling.
> She came in haste
> And most professionally set about
> Plucking the obstruction out.
> The service done she claimed her fee.
> A fee? You surely jest said he!
> You poke your neck between my jaws,
> And get it back and talk of further pay!
> Ungrateful creature! Fly away
> And take your distance from my paws.

She might see that part in herself that may at times act a little like the wolf, perhaps to a younger sibling. The fable offers the child a first and gentle awakening to her less agreeable aspects. But it would only be half the remedy if the experience were not complemented by the legend of a saint who overcomes the baser inclinations that we all fall prey to.

Stories of Saint Francis of Assisi are much loved by children of this age. His love for nature resonates deeply with the child. He sings to

Brother Sun and Sister Moon and talks to the birds; he embraces lepers and helps the poor. The story of his courageous taming of the wolf of Gubbio will not fail to have a deep impact on a child who has first heard the fable of the wolf and the stork. In this way, the separated parts become whole again, united in the child. Her soul will relate these stories to one another and she will actively find the balance between the extremes. Together, the two separate stories become incentives to achieve a wholesome inner balance.

The Authority of Scripture (age nine)

The child at the age of nine awakens to his own individuality and his own soul-life, with all the attendant possibilities of good and evil. An emerging sense of responsibility dawns on the horizon of his soul.

This makes him seek guidance. And since he cannot yet find it in himself, he will seek it from parents, mentors, family members, friends and teachers.

At this stage he longs for authority in the best sense of the word. That means true authority, authority that is followed because it is loved, respected and deeply believed in. The child at this time believes something to be true not because he can fully understand it, but because it was stated by someone he deeply respects. A statement is true because Mum or Dad or the teacher said so. The authority is the proof, not the facts. A heated discussion at this age may end with the unshakeable argument, 'It's true because my dad said so. So there!'

Many Old Testament stories meet this stage of the child. There is no need to see these stories as necessitating a commitment to Judaism or Christianity. Take them as a particular means of story medicine for a particular phase of development. (You may know other stories that will accomplish this by different means.)

The emerging individuality of the child will be attracted by the first appearance of individuality on the stage of history. The growing realization of being an 'I' will find satisfaction in the meeting with a divinity whose name is 'I am that I am'.

The dawning self, that invisible centre of the child's soul-life, will be able to relate to stories of the invisible god who leads his people through trial and tribulations. Yahweh is to the people of Israel what the child's self longs to be for his soul: a centre of reference and a strong guide.

The self will eventually be his own authority. In the meantime he needs the firm support of parents and teachers and stories that convincingly capture the spirit of authority. This will help his first unsure steps toward individuality find a strong foothold. The nine-year-old child craves form. The strict commandments and firm laws that underscore the Hebrew stories will very likely appeal to his soul.

To the modern mind this may reek of outdated authority or unwanted religiosity — not everyone wants to expose their child to the dogma of a religious faith. But this expression of outer authority may provide a much needed step towards independence from authority later on: outer authority is an important step on the ladder towards inner authority, authenticity, independent judgement, spiritual freedom and creative capability.

Education is a kind of magical ladder. The rungs we do not climb at the bottom leave a gap at the top, when we need them most. We tread in thin air and cannot progress further unless we go back and integrate the stages we have left unheeded. Coming to terms with outer authority to gain inner authenticity is best practised when it is most easy and enjoyable. (Suppressed or ignored, the desire for outer authority may rear its head in later life in the numerous Hydra masks of rational, philosophic and scientific beliefs that are as dogmatic and authoritative as a religious faith.)

I remember my stepdaughter at the age of eight or nine demanding that we write down all her household tasks as well as the consequences for not attending to them. Rules are important at this stage, and when they are clearly written down they can be clearly obeyed or broken. A child will naturally do both. In each case rules will shape the child's individuality and give him something to wrestle with.

When Jacob wrestles all night long with an angel of God, he receives in the morning the angel's blessing and is given a new name — Israel, meaning 'the one who wrestled with God.' It is not surprising therefore that the whole history of his nation became a continuous wrestling with its god.

From the very start, Jacob's tribe resisted Moses and the plans of his god. The Israelites even managed to break their covenant with Yahweh before it was fully set in stone. For a people of the law their history is uniquely unruly, and this makes for great tales. From the pious Noah, the cunning Jacob and the clever Joseph, to the headstrong and rebellious followers of Moses, the journey these stories take parallels the path of the child. Of course, the stories have to be well selected and carefully edited.

An important strength of these tales lies in their uninterrupted time-line. Folktales have the taste of eternity; they go beyond time. Fables unfold in the interior time of soul and a legend may encompass the life-time of a saint. But the biblical account stretches from the creation of the world right into historic reality. Starting with Paradise and the arche-typal figures of Adam and Eve, Cain and Abel, it goes on to immerse the imagination in the universal memory of the flood in the story of Noah's ark. Descending through the long ladder of generations we come to the historic tales of Joseph and his coat of many colours, Samson and Delilah, David and Goliath; the wisdom of King Solomon, Jonah and the whale and Daniel in the lion's den.

The biblical scriptures are the only opportunity I know of to encoun-ter a continuous myth, a story that is also history, a tale that marks all the major events of the human sojourn on earth from the creation of the world to the time of Christ. This is the unique gift of the Hebrew tradi-tion to western civilization.

Joseph and his Brothers

Of all the Bible stories, Joseph and his Brothers is possibly the most loved. It begins in the semi-paradisiacal state of Joseph's childhood. As the spoiled favourite of his father, Joseph has little care until he dreams two prophetic dreams and naively shares them with his already envious brothers.

> For, behold, we were binding sheaves in the field, and, lo, my sheaf arose, and also stood upright; and, behold, your sheaves stood round about, and made obeisance to my sheaf.
> And his brethren said to him, Shalt thou indeed reign over us? or shalt thou indeed have dominion over us? And they hated him yet the more for his dreams, and for his word.
> *Genesis 37:7-8*

The incensed brothers conspire against Joseph and eventually sell him as into slavery in Egypt. They tear his coat into pieces and convince their father that Joseph has been killed by wild animals.

In Egypt, Joseph is bought by Potiphar, captain of the pharaoh's guard. Everything prospers under Joseph's hands and he is made overseer of the captain's house. But Potiphar's wife desires Joseph. When he refuses her she makes false accusations and Joseph is put in prison. Even here his abilities make him an overseer under the keeper of the prison.

In the dungeon he meets the pharaoh's former butler and baker. Both have fallen from grace and await their sentence. Joseph interprets their dreams, and rightly foretells the butler's return to his former office and the baker's death sentence.

Two years later the pharaoh himself has two troubling dreams. He sees seven fat cows come out of the river and feed on a meadow. Then seven lean cows follow the fat cows and devour them. The next day pharaoh dreams of seven ears of good corn devoured by seven ears of thin corn.

The pharaoh summons all his magicians and wise men but none can interpret the dreams. Then the butler remembers Joseph and he is brought before the pharaoh.

Joseph interprets the dreams as indicating seven years of plenty followed by seven years of famine. Not only a man of vision, he is also a man of foresight, and knows how to make use of it.

> Now therefore let Pharaoh look out a man discreet and wise,
> and set him over the land of Egypt.
>
> Let Pharaoh do this, and let him appoint officers over the
> land, and take up the fifth part of the land of Egypt in the seven
> plenteous years.
>
> And let them gather all the food of those good years that
> come, and lay up corn under the hand of Pharaoh, and let them
> keep food in the cities.
>
> And that food shall be for store to the land against the seven
> years of famine, which shall be in the land of Egypt; that the
> land perish not through the famine.
>
> *Genesis 41:33-36*

The pharaoh is impressed and Joseph is promoted to a prominent position. All of Egypt comes under his rule and he wisely prepares during the years of plenty for the years of lack. When the great famine descends, there is grain only in Egypt and the whole world comes to buy from Joseph.

Among the many pilgrims for grain are his brothers, who have no idea of his position. Joseph has waited for this moment. He puts his brothers through severe trials and administers a good dose of story medicine, which makes them remember their guilt and repent it. Only then does he reveal himself to them. The moment of recognition and forgiveness is one the most touching episodes in literature: one can hardly refrain from weeping with Joseph and rejoicing with his brothers.

Joseph is a visionary who can translate imagination into reality, vision into thought. This is a unique gift, possessed by no one else in the whole of Egypt. The pharaoh's realm still sleeps in the imaginal powers of the past. To interpret a dream, to make sense of the imagination, requires a new capacity for intellectuality, thought, reason. Joseph is a forerunner in these. It is through them that he knows what to do: to save in the years of plenty for the years of dearth.

We are so familiar with economic planning and large organizational feats that it is easy to overlook the initiatory power of this story. In the history of humanity, Joseph is a pioneer in the rational handling of economic affairs. He is the first entrepreneur. He has what all entrepreneurs need: vision and intellect, foresight and practical ability. His combination of gifts saves Egypt and its neighbouring countries from starvation and makes Egypt rich.

Joseph is the first historic figure to have a real career, working his way from the bottom up. He starts as a slave and through his abilities ends up in the most responsible position in the known world. He is the right man in the right place.

For Joseph is not just a master of economics. He is also proficient in matters of the soul. He handles the forgiveness of his brothers in the same masterful way that he handles the wheat production of Egypt. He has a long-term vision and the patience to implement it in stages. He is motivated by forgiveness, not revenge, but he does not make it easy for his brothers. He orchestrates an elaborate trial to effect their repentance. He has learned the lessons his own destiny has taught him and he applies them to others: he puts his brothers through the same transformative ups and downs that he himself suffered and so helps them to come to terms with their guilt. Joseph is an early psychologist and his method is one of action.

Joseph is a character that children will immediately take to, particularly around nine years of age. For at that time they too have access to both imagination and intellect. The former is still alive and the latter not yet fully dominant. Like Joseph they live in both worlds and like Joseph they need to relate one to the other. The story of Joseph gives them the confidence that this is possible: that imagination and intellect, vision and rationalism, can go hand in hand, can work together. Children learn from his life that dire problems of the world and of the soul — famine and betrayal — can be solved through the marriage of intellect and imagination.

In its own time this story helped the imagination to befriend the intellect. In our time the story assists the intellect to see the lost potential of the imagination. To the child it does both.

15. The Twilight of Childhood

Norse Myth (age ten)

After the ninth year the Waldorf curriculum draws on Norse myth, a draft brewed in the cauldron of Germanic imagination. As story medicine, northern myths are purgatives. They clear away the past and make room for the new. They also serve as a fitting antidote to the omnipotent one god of the scriptures. Not only are the Nordic tales full of gods, giants, dwarves, elves, witches, Valkyries and warriors: their gods are mortal and live in constant fear of the giants and other formidable enemies such as the Fenris Wolf and the Midgard Snake. The vigorous characters of Norse myth speak to the new sense of individuality in the child.

The trickster Loki speaks to the cunning trickster that awakens at this time in them. They will love the exploits of the valiant Thor who dresses as a woman to regain his hammer from the giants, particularly the moment he takes off his veil, grabs his magic hammer and wreaks thunderous revenge. They will be deeply moved by the tragic death of the beautiful and much loved Baldur through the cunning of Loki. With Baldur's death the fate of the Norse gods is sealed.

They too look with trepidation towards the end of their world, when Loki will rise up with all his evil company to storm Valhalla. This is Ragnarok, the long prophesied Twilight of the Gods in which even Wotan, the Nordic father god, meets his end in the fangs of the Fenris Wolf.

The Germanic myth powerfully captures the death blow dealt by the rising intellect to the imagination. The death of the imaginative perception is the death of the gods. The child relives this death around the age of ten. The ten year old's crisis is the Ragnarok of childhood. Childhood ends, the imagination weakens and with it the glamour of childhood begins to fade. Wordsworth retained a vivid memory of this transition in his own life in 'Intimations of Immortality' from *Recollections of Early Childhood*:

> There was a time when meadow, grove, and stream,
> The earth, and every common sight,

To me did seem
Apparell'd in celestial light,
The glory and the freshness of a dream.
It is not now as it hath been of yore; —
Turn wheresoe'er I may,
By night or day,
The things which I have seen I now can see no more ...

Our birth is but a sleep and a forgetting:
The Soul that rises with us, our life's Star,
Hath had elsewhere its setting,
And cometh from afar:
Not in entire forgetfulness,
And not in utter nakedness,
But trailing clouds of glory do we come
From God, who is our home:
Heaven lies about us in our infancy!
Shades of the prison-house begin to close
Upon the growing Boy ...

We can see the intellect begin to creep into the mind. The warm colours vanish and a cold hue hangs over the world. Former idols shatter. The insignia of the mother-goddess is taken from Mum. The stature of Dad falls to its real size. The teacher is lowered from his pedestal of admiration. The twilight of all former gods has begun.

As all strongholds loosen, there comes a sense of insecurity and sometimes fear. Ragnarok is in process. The Fenris Wolf of the intellect strips the flesh of authority from the father god. The hissing Midgard Snake poisons the imagination with criticism and disbelief. From this moment stories become merely stories and a good part of childhood is lost in the flood of destruction. But one part survives in the animal tales popular at this age.

Animal Tales

This time it is real animal stories rather than fables. Stories that track the animal into its own habitat — the smooth life of the otter, the long journey of salmon and the migration of birds, polar bears in the arctic snow and the family of lions in the African heat. This is the moment to meet the ancient customs of elephants and dive with whales and dolphins.

While the mythical creatures such as the Fenris Wolf vanish together with the gods, the real animals of this world retain a memory of their fabulous ancestry. They are imagination incarnate: even in the age of the intellect a lion retains a measure of royalty. Children still glimpse the gold shimmering through the thick fur of a bear and dolphins cannot help but leap to the attention of the heart — as do all animals, sea creatures and birds at this age when presented in story. Such stories awaken memories of the former imaginal life, the kingdom of childhood and the old ways and carefree days lost in the tangle of pre-adolescence.

At this time horses will gallop into your child's life of their own accord, and girls will often have a whole stable of horse books. Mothers are harnessed for the weekly hunt through libraries and fathers lasso stray copies of *Black Beauty* in bookstores. When interest in other animals begins to recede in the turbulent years, the passion for horses remains. Though equipped with only four legs and not eight like Wotan's trusty Sleipnir, the imagination of the horse will carry the child in and out of Germanic myth and save them from the pervasive Ragnarok of the intellect.

The Grace of Greece (age eleven)

Waldorf education assists the transition from childhood imagination to teenage reality with a carefully orchestrated symphony of tales. Norse myth is followed by lively and graceful Greek myth in a perfect cure for the shattering Twilight of the Gods. Greek myths stand at the transition between imagination and thought, myth and history. Because of this they are ideally prefaced with the older myths of India, Persia, Egypt and Babylon. Parts of the Ramayana, of Babylonian creation myth and the stories of Isis and Osiris can be called on to meet the needs of the child. In this way myths precede history and make it palatable. The Greek myths enhance this process by leading the last remnants of childhood imagination into the first acquaintance with thought. Just like the ancient Greeks, the child at this stage strikes a rare balance between imagination and intellect.

This is the time to take in a good dose of Greek myth. The stories of Eurydice and Orpheus, Ariadne and Theseus, Perseus and Medusa, and of all the heroes in and outside of Troy — Cassandra, Penelope, the bright Hector, the quick-footed Achilles and the cunning Odysseus make fabulous tales.

From Rome to Romance (age twelve onward)

And when the intellect has taken control it is time for Roman stories. These contain almost no myth, little legend, but a lot of history. The Romans are a sober people, practical and unimaginative. Their genius exhausted itself in the creation of the republic, in complex laws, engineering feats, military tactics and clever diplomacy. Romans are ideal lawyers and politicians, just like the twelve year old who becomes politic at home — a republican ready to challenge the status quo. The rule of Mum and Dad is over. Just as in ancient Rome the old has to yield to a new constitution. Agreements have to be reached in the family senate. This is the perfect time for disagreement and discussion and carefully negotiated terms. Roman history is full of stories that match this phase.

By the end of this stage, superficiality ought to have become depth, and external bravado makes way for a greater internal feeling life. But the personality is still a mask, and behind it the face of the soul awaits discovery.

One pathway to the soul is through medieval Romance, a genre that has its origins in the most soulful of ages. Arthurian knights and ladies are the perfect introduction to this phase. They touch the soul and make it tender. The knights may be resplendent in armour, but beneath the iron skin they are as sensitive as teenagers of this age, and just as alone and lost.

The medieval knight who rides alone, suffering pangs of love in pursuit of his quest, serves as a picture for boys of this age who hide their tender self behind the armour of sunglasses and attitude.

Like a midwife, the Arthurian stories assist the birth of emotional individuality. This is an arduous journey through unfamiliar territory, best undertaken with the help of those who have been there before — explorers in the terrain of human relationships. Tristan and Iseult are the unrivalled experts on the topic of unattainable love, Arthur and Guinevere and Lancelot exemplify the complications of relationship, Sir Gawain and his lady reveal the power of transformation, and Sigune's dedication to her dead lover shows the power of unwavering love. In these stories the teenager looks into a mirror of his own tender soul. The best part in him will understand the high ideals of Dante, who dedicated his life and literary work to a girl he met at the age of nine and knew he could never hope to marry.

First love embodies in teenagers a longing for their own soul projected onto an idealized and unattainable figure. This first love is an important moment in the awakening of the soul and it is reflected in the nature of courtly love.

Unfortunately, the delicate beginnings of love are easily cut short by the omnipresent gospel of sex, of quick and easy relationships and the push and shove of lovers on the public screen. In this atmosphere the soul can be aborted before it is fully born.

The pangs of first love are the labour of this birth. Every longing stretches the soul. Every unfulfilled desire tones the emotional muscles and makes them strong. Through enduring agonies and ecstasies the soul takes shape. Every pain and every joy mark the soul's perimeter and enlarge it. First love often resurrects the imagination that was previously lost and manifests itself in love poetry. Such poems are the signature of the soul. (A diary at this time can be a safety valve, a map of the soul's journey in search of itself and a perfect place for the soul to relieve its loneliness.)

Arthurian myth and stories of troubadours offer a complete awakening into the complexities of human relationships; a teenager's guide towards emotional authenticity. Once this authenticity is gained, the soul is anchored. It has found the safety of harbour. From the safety of harbour it can sail forth into unknown continents.

Uncharted Territory

Puberty is an age of exploration. For the ardent reader, it can be matched by the age of exploration that followed medieval times. The European explorers found their way through uncharted territory. Like teenagers, they lacked maps, but drew them themselves.

The teenager encounters great biographies in the destinies of explorers like Vasco de Gama and Francis Drake. Henry the Seafarer and Christopher Columbus go against the grain of public opinion. They embody the independent spirit and break the paradigms that limit the horizon of their world. This is the time to meet the self-willed Eleanor of Aquitaine and the courageous Saint Joan.

Like Columbus, teenagers are driven to meet the world and change it, to entertain fresh thoughts and daring ideas, to break new ground, challenge the boundaries, go further than anybody else has dared to go, beyond the world-view of the parents, to find a new world and a new life within it. Puberty is a passionate time, a time of enthusiasm.

The history of exploration widened the horizon of the world. Now the history of science widens the horizon of the mind. From the perspective of story medicine, science is not the exploration of fact but the exploration of the human mind. Galileo and Copernicus saw the same facts their predecessors saw for thousands of years, but they saw them differently.

Copernicus is famed for changing the model of the world by putting the sun (not the earth) at the centre of the universe. He ought to be even more famous for changing the status of the human mind. Telling a new story about the old tale he proved that we can see things differently. He put the mind at the centre of the universe and made all meaning revolve around it. He was postmodern centuries before it became fashionable. Like all teenagers, Copernicus was a revolutionary. He sowed the seed of individual freedom long before it became political reality. He was a pioneer of the self-reliant personality that every teenager aspires to.

In this revolutionary science, physics was the playground of the intellect, a solid mirror for the ephemerals of the modern mind and the inquiry into oneself. Science was not what it seemed. Behind its surface of facts hid the most human of enterprise, the search for the self, the quest for self-knowledge. Copernicus and Kepler, Galileo and Bruno began this quest. Every discovery and every new insight had to be fought for against resistance. Giordano Bruno ended on the stake. Galileo spent years under house arrest. Others suffered poverty or ridicule, but all stood by their search for truth. In this way, they transformed our culture.

The stories of these lives, which combined vision with the power of thought, inspire confidence in the future and in the human capacity to make sense of the world. They inspire faith that new meanings can be discovered and an old story can change into a new tale. They remind us that science has a human side and that even the most complex of machines is made by the mind. Through their biographies the teenager comes to know all the strengths they so urgently need to discover themselves, to formulate goals and ground their visions in the reality of this world.

16. New Tales for Old

Myth and folktale are more often authored by a people than an individual. They are part of the shared imagination of the past. By contrast, new stories have a traceable author. They are the creation of individual effort.

The deliberate making of imaginative tales can be traced to the Romantics. While the Brothers Grimm collected the old stories, poets like Goethe and Novalis began to create new tales. Initially, these creations were aimed at the imaginatively gifted adult — a poet's gift to those poetically inclined. Later, the tales of Hans Christian Anderson and Oscar Wilde were directed more towards the child and sparked a whole genre of children's literature in their wake.

Writers like C.S. Lewis and Tolkien, Phillip Pullman, Michael Ende and J.K. Rowling have elevated the imaginative tale into an art form. As fantasy their tales are able to be real in a higher sense and can introduce themes that might otherwise be anathema. These stories are powerful medicine and have to be handled with care: used at the right moment.

Children need guidance into the adventurous realm of contemporary myth. Tolkien's *Lord of the Rings* is the first true epic of the modern imagination and a masterpiece of English. But though it is a signpost of hope for the imaginative tale, it has to be used with care. *The Hobbit* is fine for a ten year old, but *Lord of the Rings* is not. While it is a good read for teenagers, it is a 'grown up' myth, too dark and complex for a young child.

Ideally children's stories come with a guide to age-appropriateness. Authors often give this unconsciously, in the age of the heroes that populate their tales: Harry Potter is exactly eleven when he is invited to join Hogwarts' school of magic. Milne's Christopher Robin is pre-school age, and Ende's Bastian Balthazar Bux is about nine when he embarks on his Never Ending Story.

Harry Potter

I am in two minds about Rowling's creation, particularly as literature for young children. I think the books and films are often encountered too early. Harry Potter is great fantasy, but a certain foundation of soul needs to be established before a child enters the gothic labyrinth of Hogwarts.

The Potter books are based on the mystery novel and the emotional suspense created by this genre. In most mystery novels we do not know who the murderer is until the very end. In the Harry Potter books, the murder is yet to come. Though we know it is the Dark Lord who is attempting to kill Harry, we do not know under which mask he is hiding. This makes the books even more harrowing for the soul than conventional mysteries.

The dark forces in the Harry Potter series are hidden and unscrupulous, and ever more brilliant as the books progress. The portrayal of evil echoes the racial ethos of the Nazi regime and procedures of black magic. All this may be exciting and highly stimulating reading for the imagination-deprived teenager, but it is not appropriate for younger readers, who need to know who is good and who is bad so they can morally orientate themselves in a story.

In fairytales, evil and cruelty are dealt with imaginatively. The wolf that devours Red Riding Hood spills no blood and the child is soon revived. But the killing in Harry Potter is real and irreversible. The blood that is spilled is 'real' blood that will leave a mark on a young child's soul. The cruelty of a sinister figure like Voldemort is too convincing to be digested before a child is equipped to face him. Too young, they may fall prey to his schemes — and as the book tells you, he is eager to kill them as young as he can.

I recommend you to the advice of the world expert in all matters concerning Harry Potter and the care of the magical and endangered child: Albertus Dumbledore, Director of Hogwarts School of Magic. The wise Professor protected Harry from all contact with the shady and dangerous world of magic until he had reached the age of eleven. I take this as the story's own explicit advice for its appropriate use: children should reach this age before being admitted to the school of sorcery.

I have said I am in two minds about Harry Potter. While I am concerned about its premature use, it nevertheless provides a good dose of fantasy for teenage consumption. It also speaks directly to contemporary myth — its popularity shows that the stories answer a dire need in our culture: the story deprivation of contemporary childhood.

Children recognise themselves in Harry. Like the modern child he starts off deprived of imagination and magic, denied his birthright to be an adventurer in any realm other than this world. Like the modern child he is endowed with imaginal gifts and has been brought up by parents who are 'muggles' — totally unmagical folk. Most parents are 'Dursleys,' not only lacking imagination, they suppress it with any means at their disposal.

The imaginal part in every modern child is as maltreated by parents and education as Harry Potter is by the Dursleys, while the child's conventional and unmagical part is as spoiled as his stepbrother Dudley — who is the very kind of insensitive and competitive bully our world seems to reward while the Harrys are locked in the closets and punished for who they are.

Harry Potter exemplifies the drama of the imaginative child. This is what makes his story a modern myth. He is the hero who escapes the prison of convention, breaking through the brick walls of King's Cross Station into a new dimension of imaginal adventure. Harry is a symbol for the imaginal child and her adventures in this world and the next — but for a young child there are smoother ways to break the brick walls of convention. A new dimension may be more easily entered through an old wardrobe hung with fur coats.

The Chronicles of Narnia

C.S. Lewis's *Chronicles of Narnia* are a masterpiece of children's literature. A nine year old can appreciate the imaginative treasures this series contains, and there is no need to censor their use, for the stories have a purity that will protect them from misuse. The children who are the heroes of many of the Narnia tales are aged between seven and twelve, and that seems a good indication of their age-appropriateness.

The *Chronicles of Narnia* are story medicine at its best. Whenever I am recovering from sickness I read a Narnia book and find they work better than vitamins. They stabilize the soul and through the soul, the body.

When you embark on the Narnia stories you are in familiar territory, and so is the child. Each tale is a homecoming to one or another province of the soul — it maps an adventure that calls for the great-hearted heroism of a lion. Children who hear that call are transformed. The traitor, Edmund, becomes King Edmund the First; the notorious Eustace Clarence Scrubb sheds his dragon skin and becomes the likeable hero of further adventures. And just as the heroes of the Narnia books are profoundly changed by their encounter with Aslan the great lion, so are the readers.

Harry Potter is fantasy with mythological elements. The *Chronicles of Narnia* are much stronger myth, a product of exact imagination, revealing realities beyond the apparently real. The Narnia stories meet the soul on its own home ground. They speak the imaginative language of the heart and carry the power of transformation that only this language can provide.

It is this transformative capacity that Harry Potter lacks. He is a likeable hero and remains so, even as he becomes more adept in magic. He is protected by the love of his mother, but he is not touched by the love that changes the heart. He remains a somewhat superficial hero, the master of outer accomplishment and victories. He is Superboy equipped with magical powers and all the gadgets of the trade: owls and broomsticks, invisibility cloak and miraculous maps.

Momo and the Neverending Story

Michael Ende's *Neverending Story* is an epic of children's literature, a rich feast for the imagination. It contains the very map that makes a superficial hero into a real one. Its hero, Bastian Balthazar Bux, enters the imaginal realm of Fantasia by means of a magical book. The story is complex and is true story medicine — much of what I have said in these pages is said there too by imaginative means and clothed in an adventure that is a depth account of the soul's journey towards integration. In this journey the headstrong Medusa of unbridled fantasy is turned into an imagination with a heart.

The *Neverending Story* is the length of an epic. If you do not have the time for such long stories, read Ende's *Momo and the Grey Gentlemen* instead. This is an important book for children and adults, one that ought to be read and performed in schools and theatres, in hospitals and city parks. It is a true modern myth and offers story medicine for the most widespread epidemic of our civilization: the lack of time. Once you have read *Momo* you will *make* time for the *Neverending Story.*

Momo contains a message for everyone, even for young children, perhaps especially for them. It is, however, not written to suit the pre-school age. But fortunately, there is another story that is, and one which will achieve something similar — A.A. Milne's *Winnie the Pooh.*

Winnie the Pooh

Winnie the Pooh is *Momo* in bear format. Pooh always has time and is never rushed. In his home it is always eleven o'clockish and just the right moment for a little something, which is either honey or honey. Pooh lives in sweet time. He embodies the comfort and benevolence of the bear in all of us. *Winnie the Pooh* is inspired by the genius of English childhood itself. We immediately feel at home with Eeyore and Piglet, Rabbit and Kanga. They are our friends as much as Pooh's. To the child, they are an extended family of imaginary companions.

Winnie the Pooh is the perfect complement to fairytales. The little adventures, the humour, the poetry and the good-natured spirit that pervades the books, speak directly to the child. While fairytales explore the interior of the soul, *Winnie the Pooh* captures childhood imagination in its transition to reality. The stories are a gentle guide to the world beyond childhood and contain a brilliant introduction to the temperaments that begin to assert themselves by school age: Eeyore is melancholy incarnate; Rabbit is choleric; Roo exemplifies the buoyant sanguinity of the young child. Pooh is not only the 'best of bears' but the best that the phlegmatic temperament has to offer — the benevolent friend and trusty companion through the childhood of the imagination.

All this makes *Winnie the Pooh* a timeless classic, a *Neverending Story* in is own right that can be enjoyed at any age, reading it again or hearing it on audio tape. Unlike the intimate fairytale, it offers itself to this medium, which can be a great help on long car trips and plane flights and even at home. The same is true of other stories that follow in the wake of *Winnie the Pooh. The Wind in the Willows* will capture the child's imagination for a long time with the amiable water rat and mole, the hardy badger and the marvellously conceited and totally adorable toad.

Winnie the Pooh and *Wind in the Willows* can accompany the child until the imagination closes around the age of nine or so. It is then that the portals to Narnia can open it again. The best children's stories resurrect the imagination from the intellectual assault of this world. They are more than remedies. They are life savers that preserve the child's creative forces from premature death.

Teenage Fiction

Going into puberty, novels like Harry Potter or Susan Cooper's *The Dark is Rising* can be followed by more mature works. Some of the novels written for the age group of thirteen to fifteen ascend to a level of artistry that captivates adults and teenagers alike, among them Ursula Le Guin's *Wizard of Earthsea* and Madeleine L'Engle's *A Wrinkle in Time*.

The *Wizard of Earthsea* is a masterpiece hero quest, one of the great transformational tales that treats the remote past and early magic with an authenticity that only a great writer can achieve.

Madeleine L'Engle's *Wrinkle in Time* explores the imaginal dimension of science when the child heroes of her novel are hurled into a future pervaded by inhuman technology and mass manipulation. Through the power of love they overcome the brain-machine masterminding the technological universe and so save the world from an inhuman future. This is more than a good novel. It is a prophetic book that captures the essence of science fiction writing. Every science fiction novel is a wrinkle in time. It confronts us with the dangers of an overly technological world and asks us whether this is the kind of civilization we want to create.

One important way to help create a more human future lies in the making of new tales. For those who wish to take this path the third part of this book offers a map that will help their imagination to take the necessary steps.

Part 3. The Making of Stories

17. Poetic Birth & the Tale of Taliesin

Through parenting my son I became a storyteller and story-maker. I soon realized that it is good to tell a traditional tale and even better to create a new story. In the first case the imagination is greatly stimulated, in the second it comes truly alive.

The more I practised the more I came to see the spontaneous telling of stories as an alchemical art in which the storyteller and the hero face similar trials. Like their heroes, story-makers leave the familiar ground of the known, the security of established tales and premeditated plots. They put all their trust in the new, the unknown and unexpected.

The storyteller's daring in exploring the continents of unknown tales gives their child listeners the bravery to face the world. For storytelling takes courage to reach out to the new, the immediate and utterly present. Uncertainty is always creative.

If you are a parent, practise on children — they are your best audience. They know that a fresh tale comes straight from the heart. They relish the moments of imaginal bonding, the meeting with what is most creative in us — that part in ourselves that is as young as the heart: for it is there that the spontaneous story creates itself in the moment it is told.

I recommend the same attitude to all story-makers, no matter whether they have an immediate audience or not. Though writing a story is not as spontaneous an act as telling one, it can be made so. All it takes is to bravely enter into the act of creation and forgo all premeditated plots. This will make your writing as adventurous as the stories you tell.

Most of the stories in this part of the book were written in this way. Some students wrote them with a particular child in mind; others used the exercises to stimulate their imagination to produce good stories.

This book wishes to serve both purposes — to provide guidelines that will enable real children to receive the stories they need and a manual for story-makers to nourish their inner child and help it become creative. For the sake of simplicity I will hereon conceive of the reader as a parent and assume that all story-makers are parents in a wider sense.

The Developing Imagination

The daily telling of stories to my son inspired me to explore this art further and I began to look for pathways to stimulate the imagination. I found them in the steps that the imagination itself takes in the growing child.

The imagination is born in stages. Before the age of three the forces of the imagination are closely bound up with the body. The Herculean labour of bodily growth consumes all mental activity. During this time the child still lives in an animated world. The next chapter helps the story-maker to access this world by means of the doll.

The following two chapters lead from the animated world of the early years to the world that we know. 'Taming Place and Time' and 'Coming to the Senses' address this stage and help the child to orientate himself in his new environment. The story-making suggestions in these chapters are pertinent to children aged between two and four.

After the third year the imagination is slowly released into activity. This takes place in stages and proceeds slowly. Between the age of three and five the imagination is largely stimulated by outside events. If you watch children play at this time you will observe that their imagination is stimulated by any object they come across. A piece of wood becomes a truck or train. At this stage stories can be used to prompt the imagination in the same way that objects do. This is the time for the storyteller to start to draw on the imaginal allies and elemental beings described in Chapters Twenty-one and Twenty-two. The two chapters that follow take the use of these allies deeper and further through the use of metaphor.

After the age of five the imagination becomes increasingly motivated from within. If you watch children play at this time you will find that their ideas now precede the outer object. An inner centre of initiative is discovered and the hero of the soul is born, a hero who longs for stories to match his state. The development of these stories is described in Chapter Twenty-five, 'The Laboratory of the Imagination.' Once you have learned to distil your hero from the retort of the imagination, the complete art of story-making is well within reach.

Following the imagination in this way provides a secure, organic, step-by-step process that develops the imaginal capacity according to its own laws. The process can be easily used by parents, teachers and counsellors to help a child with the appropriate medicinal story. Of course any story-maker can benefit from following these steps to gain creative momentum.

The Child's World

Our stories have to meet the soul in order that their full potential should unfold. They must be on familiar terrain and feel like old acquaintances. Such stories will assure the child that his own way of experiencing the world is understood by those around him and so validate his way of being.

To match story with child we need to know the state of his soul. To do this we need to entertain a totally different way of experiencing the world — a state most of us forgot the moment we first said 'I.' This was the moment we left the paradise of childhood, when we began to distinguish ourselves from the world: the moment we began to divide the world into me and you, mine and yours, here and there, in and out.

The very young child has not entered the unfamiliar terrain of this world fully. He is still hovering in his own cocoon of experience. But what world does the child inhabit? To answer this question let us listen to the great tale of the Welsh bard Taliesin.

> The sorceress Ceridwen is much grieved by the ugly looks of her ill-favoured son Mordred. To make up for her son's misfortune she resolves to make him into a great bard by means of a magical potion.
>
> She orders a large cauldron to be heated and kept boiling for the space of a year. She gathers rare herbs and with many incantations she casts them into the brew. A servant boy named Gwion is appointed to stir the brew and guard it while she is away. For Ceridwen knew that only the first drop tasted of the potion would impart the power and all-knowing of a bard.
>
> On the very last day Ceridwen left again to gather one more herb. She orders Gwion to guard the pot with special care.
>
> Gwion kept the fire going and stirred with all his might. The cauldron hissed and bubbled and one hot drop of the magic brew spurted on his thumb. Pained by the sudden burn, Gwion stuck his thumb into his mouth and so tasted the brew.
>
> At that very moment all the power and knowledge of all the ancient bards descended on Gwion.
>
> By his new-gained powers he knew that Ceridwen would soon seek revenge for her thwarted plans. And so he fled as fast as his young legs would carry him. But Ceridwen soon knew what had happened and followed him apace.

As fast as he ran, she ran faster. When Gwion, using his new-won power, changed himself into a hare, Ceridwen changed into a greyhound. And as fast as he ran she ran faster. At a river Gwion changed into a fish. But Ceridwen became an otter. And as fast as he swam she swam faster. Gwion leapt from the water and became a bird. But Ceridwen became a hawk. And as fast as he flew, she flew faster. And again and again he shifted his shape. But again and again Ceridwen followed him.

Finally Gwion saw a pile of wheat and he hid himself in a single grain. But Ceridwen turned into a speckled hen and with a keen eye found the grain and swallowed it whole.

But this was not to be the end of Gwion. For Ceridwen soon found herself pregnant and as she had lain with no man she knew that the child she carried under her bosom was none other than Gwion. Then she and her ugly son Mordred conspired to kill the baby as soon as it was born.

But when the time had come and the baby was born, it was of such radiant beauty that Ceridwen could not kill him. To save the child from the envious Mordred she sewed him into a little leather bag and set him adrift on the ocean.

Not long thereafter the young prince Elphin, fishing for salmon in his father's weir, found the heavy bundle in his nets. Disappointed not to have caught any salmon, Elphin opened the bag and to his great surprise found a baby. He called *out* 'Taliesin' which in the old Welsh tongue means 'radiant brow'. And to his even greater surprise the baby replied.

> Yes Taliesin that is my name
> Fair Elphin do not lament the lack of salmon
> No catch was ever as good as today
> Fair Elphin be of good cheer
> Though I am small I am skilful
> And will bring you good luck
> There are wonders on my tongue
> And my help will be with you
> Whenever you are in need.

How is it that a baby can talk? marvelled Elphin, and Taliesin, already a bard, replied:

Once I was a handsome youth
Tutored in the hall of Ceridwen
Though I was small in stature
I was great in her sacred house.
She held me her prisoner
But inspiration set me free
Learned I grew in ancient laws
And in the speech before words
For the wisdom I gained
I had to flee from her hall
From the anger of Ceridwen
Her terrible call of revenge
I fled and shifted my shape.
Since then I have been a hare
And the shape of a crow
And a green frog in a pond
And high with the roe-bucks
I have leapt over thickets barring my way
I have been a raven of prophetic speech
A cunning fox, a sure swift and
A squirrel hiding in vain.
I have been the red deer
And hot iron hammered in fire
I have been the keen edge of a sword
And the cry in the midst of battle
I have been a struggling bull,
a bristling boar caught in a ravine
I have been a grain of wheat
and was eaten and born again
Put in a bag I floated on the sea
I know I have come to light again.

The young Lord Elphin takes Taliesin into his house. Once
grown to adulthood Taliesin became the most famous of bards,
a master druid and great advisor to his king. He saved his Lord
Elphin from many a trouble and brought good fortune to him
and his house.

Two features in this tale cast light on the child in its early years. The first is that the babe not only speaks but immediately utters poetry, as befits a bard and druid. Taliesin is the Welsh Merlin. The words Taliesin and Merlin both mean chief druid, high priest and initiate, an office which in the Celtic tradition is allied with the power of the word, the ability to utter poetry and make stories.

Stories about speaking babes are by no means restricted to the Welsh tradition. Jesus, Krishna and Zarathustra each spoke as soon as he was born. Buddha took four strides immediately after his birth, announcing to all four directions of the world that this was his last incarnation in the world of semblance.

The second thing that strikes us in the story of Taliesin is that he has been many things — a hare, a crow, a frog, a roebuck, a raven of prophetic speech, a fox, a swift, a sword blade, a battle-cry, a grain of wheat and much more. In short he has been everything.

Here the myth allows us to see into the world of the child and, beyond that, the childhood of humanity. The tale opens the gate of paradise, the place in time long before the division into here and there, you and me.

This is the world before separation, in which all things are one. There is nothing outside and no things yet. Whatever is — the hare, the roebuck, the sword blade — is of the same nature as the child: a being among beings.

Once we were all in this state. We shared in the undiluted essence of cat and deer and bird. To the Gnostics this was the initial state of the soul, a state in which the tree of knowledge had not yet cast its shadow on the primal light.

In this state there is only being. Being aware of is the same as being one with. Early humanity was immersed in this state and remembers it through the various myths of paradise. The young child echoes this state, first in its relationship with the mother and later and to a lesser degree through its oneness with the world.

In this world of pure being everything *is* itself: everything emanates itself, reveals itself, speaks itself. It is a thoroughly speaking world in which nothing is hidden. Whatever we encounter in this world is what we are. Taliesin remembers this world as a child and he testifies to it when he tells Elphin all he has been.

All children partake of this world in their early years, but they do so unconsciously and it is later forgotten. The stories of Taliesin, Krishna, Zarathustra and other heroes of the inner life show that they consciously remember an experience that the rest of us usually forget: the world in which all beings speak. This world still echoes in fairytales through their magical talking beasts. Taliesin and others who inhabit this world consciously exercise the power of primal speech.

> Learned I grew in ancient laws
> and in the speech before words.

This speech before words is the vernacular of all beings. It is the original mother tongue, the language of paradise, and of the world that all children leave behind when they pass through the gate of consciousness. It is a world that few adults care to re-enter. Those who do so are the mystics and saints of the various traditions. A mystic consciously inhabits the world that the child inhabits unconsciously, as expressed in the words of the Christ: 'Unless you become like little children you cannot enter the kingdom of heaven.'

T.S. Eliot captures the dynamic of this process in the closing lines of his *Four Quartets*.

> We shall not cease from exploration
> And the end of all our exploring
> Will be to arrive where we started
> And know the place for the first time ...

Eliot knew that beginning and ending wrap a world of being, communication and communion. This world is as familiar to the child as it is strange to most adults. If we want to meet the child on familiar ground, we need to enter this world. It is not easy. But luckily the wisdom of the past has produced a means by which even a sober adult may temporarily bridge the gap of separation — the doll.

18. The Magical Doll

The doll is the last echo of the world of talking creatures that even adults can hear. For adults it is a remnant of their own childhood and the last object they easily animate. Through the doll they unconsciously remember what they have forgotten: the speaking world and their childhood.

Most adults have, like the Sleeping Beauty, pricked themselves on the sharp spindle of the intellect. Their childhood memories are sleeping behind an impenetrable hedge of thorns.

Through the doll this world awakens again. She opens the door, if temporarily, to the adult's lost childhood. The doll loosens our tied-down tongue and reminds us of the first language, the language of paradise that makes everything come to life. When she speaks the world responds — soft toys and pets join the conversation and mute things find their voice.

And that is not all. Dolls also serve as soul-guides and catalysts of story medicine. To rightly understand the full potential of the doll is a necessity for both the story-maker and the conscious parent. We can gain such an understanding through a most powerful story, the Russian fairytale of Vasilissa the Beautiful.

Vasilissa the Beautiful

In a certain kingdom, across three times nine kingdoms,
beyond high mountain chains, there once lived a merchant.
He had been married for twelve years, but in that time there
had been born to him only one child, a daughter, who from the
cradle was called Vasilissa the Beautiful.

When the little girl was eight years old the mother fell ill,
and before many days it was plain to be seen that she must
die. So she called her little daughter to her, and taking a tiny
wooden doll from under the blanket of the bed, put it into her
hands and said, 'My little Vasilissa, my dear daughter, listen to
what I say, remember well my last words and fail not to carry
out my wishes. I am dying, and with my blessing, I leave to

thee this little doll. It is very precious for there is no other like
it in the whole world. Carry it always about with thee in thy
pocket and never show it to anyone. When evil threatens thee
or sorrow befalls thee, go into a corner, take it from thy pocket
and give it something to eat and drink. It will eat and drink a
little, and then thou may tell it thy trouble and ask its advice,
and it will tell thee how to act in thy time of need.' So saying,
she kissed her little daughter on the forehead, blessed her, and
shortly after she died.

Little Vasilissa grieved greatly for her mother, and her sorrow was so deep that when the dark night came, she lay in her
bed and wept and did not sleep. At length she thought of the
tiny doll, so she rose and took it from the pocket of her gown
and finding a piece of wheat bread and a cup of kvass, she set
them before it, and said, 'There, my little doll, take it. Eat a
little, and drink a little, and listen to my grief. My dear mother
is dead and I am lonely for her.'

Then the doll's eyes began to shine like fireflies, and suddenly it became alive. It ate a morsel of the bread and took
a sip of the kvass, and when it had eaten and drunk, it said,
'Don't weep, little Vasilissa. Grief is worst at night. Lie down,
shut thine eyes, comfort thyself and go to sleep. The morning
is wiser than the evening.' So Vasilissa the Beautiful lay down,
comforted herself and went to sleep, and the next day her
grieving was not so deep and her tears were less bitter.

Now after the death of his wife, the merchant sorrowed for
many days, but at the end of that time he began to desire to
marry again and to look about him for a suitable wife. This
was not difficult to find, for he had a fine house, with a stable
of swift horses, besides being a good man who gave much
to the poor. Of all the women he saw, however, the one who
suited him best of all, was a widow of about his own age with
two daughters of her own, and she, he thought, besides being
a good housekeeper, would be a kind foster mother to his little
Vasilissa.

So the merchant married the widow and brought her home
as his wife, but the little girl soon found that her foster mother
was very far from being what her father had thought. She was
a cold, cruel woman, who had desired the merchant for the

sake of his wealth, and had no love for his daughter. Vasilissa
was the greatest beauty in the whole village, while her own
daughters were as spare and homely as two crows, and because of this all three envied and hated her. They gave her all
sorts of errands to run and difficult tasks to perform, in order
that the toil might make her thin and worn and that her face
might grow brown from sun and wind, and they treated her
so cruelly as to leave few joys in life for her. But all this the
little Vasilissa endured, and while the stepmother's daughters
grew thinner and uglier, in spite of the fact that they had no
hard tasks to do, never went out in cold or rain, and sat always
with their arms folded like ladies of the Court, she herself had
cheeks like blood and milk and grew every day more beautiful.

Now the reason for this was the tiny doll, without whose
help little Vasilissa could never have managed to do all the
work that was laid upon her. Each night, when everyone else
was sound asleep, she would get up from her bed, take the doll
into a closet and, locking the door, give it something to eat and
drink, and say, 'There, my little doll, take it. Eat a little, drink
a little, and listen to my grief. I live in my father's house, but
my spiteful stepmother wishes to drive me out of the white
world. Tell me! How shall I act, and what shall I do?'

Then the little doll's eyes would begin to shine like glow-
worms, and it would become alive. It would eat a little food,
and sip a little drink, and then it would comfort her and tell
her how to act. While Vasilissa slept, it would get ready all
her work for the next day, so that she had only to rest in the
shade and gather flowers, for the doll would have the kitchen
garden weeded, and the beds of cabbage watered, and plenty
of fresh water brought from the well, and the stoves heated
exactly right. And, besides this, the little doll told her how to
make, from a certain herb, an ointment to prevent her from being sunburnt. So all the joy that came to Vasilissa came to her
through the tiny doll that she always carried in her pocket.

Years passed, till Vasilissa grew up and became of an age
when it is good to marry. All the young men in the village,
high and low, rich and poor, asked for her hand, while not one
of them stopped even to look at the stepmother's two daughters, so ill-favoured were they. This angered their mother still

more against Vasilissa; she answered every gallant who came
with the same words, 'Never shall the younger be wed before
the older ones!' and each time she let a suitor out of the door,
she would soothe her anger by beating her stepdaughter. So
while Vasilissa grew each day more lovely and graceful, she
was often miserable, and but for the little doll in her pocket,
would have longed to leave the world.

Now there came a time when it became necessary for the
merchant to leave his home and to travel to a distant kingdom.
He bade farewell to his wife and her two daughters, kissed
Vasilissa and gave her his blessing and departed, bidding them
say a prayer each day for his safe return. Scarce was he out
of sight of the village, however, when his wife sold his house,
packed all his goods and moved with them to another dwelling
far from the town, in a gloomy neighbourhood on the edge of
a wild forest. Here every day, while her two daughters were
working indoors, the merchant's wife would send Vasilissa on
one errand or other into the forest, to find a branch of a certain
rare bush or to bring her flowers or berries.

Now deep in this forest, as the stepmother well knew, there
was a green lawn and on the lawn stood a miserable little hut
on hens' legs, where lived a certain Baba Yaga, an old witch.
She lived alone and none dared go near the hut, for she ate
people as one eats chickens. The merchant's wife sent Vasilissa into the forest each day, hoping she might meet the old
witch and be devoured; but always the girl came home safe
and sound, because the little doll showed her where the flowers
and berries grew, and did not let her go near the hut that stood
on hens' legs. And each time the stepmother hated her more
because she came to no harm.

One autumn evening the merchant's wife called the three
girls to her and gave them each a task. One of her daughters
she bade make a piece of lace, the other to knit a pair of hose,
and to Vasilissa she gave a basket of flax to be spun. She bade
each finish a certain amount. Then she put out all the fires in
the house, leaving only a single candle lighted in the room
where the three girls worked, and she herself went to sleep.

They worked an hour, they worked two hours, they worked
three hours, when one of the elder daughters took up the tongs

to straighten the wick of the candle. She pretended to do this awkwardly (as her mother had bidden her) and put the candle out, as if by accident.

'What are we to do now?' asked her sister. 'The fires are all out, there is no other light in all the house, and our tasks are not done.'

'We must go and fetch fire,' said the first. 'The only house near is a hut in the forest, where a Baba Yaga lives. One of us must go and borrow fire from her.'

'I have enough light from my steel pins,' said the one who was making the lace, 'I will not go.'

'And I have plenty of light from my silver needles,' said the other, who was knitting the hose, 'and I will not go.'

'Thou, Vasilissa,' they both said, 'shall go and fetch the fire, for thou hast neither steel pins nor silver needles and cannot see to spin thy flax!' They rose up, pushed Vasilissa out of the house and locked the door, crying, 'Thou shalt not come in till thou hast fetched the fire.'

Vasilissa sat down on the doorstep, took the tiny doll from one pocket and from another the supper she had ready for it, put the food before it and said, 'There, my little doll, take it. Eat a little and listen to my sorrow. I must go to the hut of the old Baba Yaga in the dark forest to borrow some fire and I fear she will eat me. Tell me! What shall I do?'

Then the doll's eyes began to shine like two stars and it became alive. It ate a little and said, 'Do not fear, little Vasilissa. Go where thou hast been sent. While I am with thee no harm shall come to thee from the old witch.' So Vasilissa put the doll back into her pocket, crossed herself and started out into the dark, wild forest.

Whether she walked a short way or a long way the telling is easy, but the journey was hard. The wood was very dark, and she could not help trembling from fear. Suddenly she heard the sound of a horse's hoofs and a man on horseback galloped past her. He was dressed all in white, the horse under him was milk-white and the harness was white, and just as he passed her it became twilight.

She went a little further and again she heard the sound of a horse's hoofs and there came another man on horseback galloping past her. He was dressed all in red, and the horse under him was blood-red and its harness was red, and just as he passed her the sun rose.

That whole day Vasilissa walked, for she had lost her way. She could find no path in the dark wood and she had no food to set before the little doll to make it alive.

But at evening she came all at once to the green lawn where the wretched little hut stood on its hens' legs. The wall around the hut was made of human bones and on its top were skulls. There was a gate in the wall, whose hinges were the bones of human feet and whose locks were jaw-bones set with sharp teeth. The sight filled Vasilissa with horror and she stopped as still as a post buried in the ground.

As she stood there a third man on horseback came galloping up. His face was black, he was dressed all in black, and the horse he rode was coal-black. He galloped up to the gate of the hut and disappeared there as if he had sunk through the ground and at that moment the night came and the forest grew dark.

But it was not dark on the green lawn, for instantly the eyes of all the skulls on the wall were lighted up and shone till the place was as bright as day. When she saw this Vasilissa trembled so with fear that she could not run away.

Then suddenly the wood became full of a terrible noise; the trees began to groan, the branches to creak and the dry leaves to rustle, and the Baba Yaga came flying from the forest. She was riding in a great iron mortar and driving it with the pestle, and as she came she swept away her trail behind her with a kitchen broom.

She rode up to the gate and stopping, said, 'Little House, little House, stand the way thy mother placed thee, turn thy back to the forest and thy face to me!'

And the little hut turned facing her and stood still. Then smelling all around her, she cried: 'Foo! Foo! I smell a smell that is Russian. Who is here?'

Vasilissa, in great fright, came nearer to the old woman and bowing very low, said, 'It is only Vasilissa, grandmother. My stepmother's daughters sent me to thee to borrow some fire.'

'Well,' said the old witch, 'I know them. But if I give thee the fire thou shalt stay with me some time and do some work to pay for it. If not, thou shalt be eaten for my supper.' Then she turned to the gate and shouted, 'Ho! Ye, my solid locks, unlock! Thou, my stout gate, open!' Instantly the locks unlocked, the gate opened of itself, and the Baba Yaga rode in whistling. Vasilissa entered behind her and immediately the gate shut again and the locks snapped tight.

When they had entered the hut the old witch threw herself down on the stove, stretched out her bony legs and said, 'Come, fetch and put on the table at once everything that is in the oven. I am hungry.' So Vasilissa ran and lighted a splinter of wood from one of the skulls on the wall and took the food from the oven and set it before her. There was enough cooked meat for three strong men. She brought also from the cellar kvass, honey, and red wine, and the Baba Yaga ate and drank the whole, leaving the girl only a little cabbage soup, a crust of bread and a morsel of suckling pig.

When her hunger was satisfied the old witch, growing drowsy, lay down on the stove and said, 'Listen to me well, and do what I bid thee. Tomorrow when I drive away, do thou clean the yard, sweep the floors and cook my supper. Then take a quarter of a measure of wheat from my store house and pick out of it all the black grains and the wild peas. Mind thou dost all that I have bade; if not, thou shalt be eaten for my supper.'

Presently the Baba Yaga turned toward the wall and began to snore and Vasilissa knew that she was fast asleep. Then she went into the corner, took the tiny doll from her pocket, put before it a bit of bread and a little cabbage soup that she had saved, burst into tears and said, 'There, my little doll, take it. Eat a little, drink a little, and listen to my grief. Here I am in the house of the old witch and the gate in the wall is locked and I am afraid. She has given me a difficult task and if I do not do all she has bade, she will eat me tomorrow. Tell me, what shall I do?'

Then the eyes of the little doll began to shine like two candles. It ate a little of the bread and drank a little of the soup and said, 'Do not be afraid, Vasilissa the Beautiful. Be comforted. Say thy prayers, and go to sleep. The morning is wiser than the evening.' So Vasilissa trusted the little doll and was comforted. She said her prayers, lay down on the floor and went fast asleep.

When she woke next morning, very early, it was still dark.
She rose and looked out of the window, and she saw that
the eyes of the skulls on the wall were growing dim. As she
looked, the man dressed all in white, riding the milk-white
horse, galloped swiftly around the corner of the hut, leaped the
wall and disappeared, and as he went, it became quite light and
the eyes of the skulls flickered and went out. The old witch
was in the yard; now she began to whistle and the great iron
mortar and pestle and the kitchen broom flew out of the hut
to her. As she got into the mortar the man dressed all in red,
mounted on the blood-red horse, galloped like the wind around
the corner of the hut, leaped the wall and was gone, and at that
moment the sun rose. Then the Baba Yaga shouted, 'Ho! Ye,
my solid locks, unlock! Thou, my stout gate, open!' And the
locks unlocked and the gate opened and she rode away in the
mortar, driving with the pestle and sweeping away her path
behind her with the broom.

When Vasilissa found herself left alone, she examined the
hut, wondering to find it filled with such an abundance of
everything. Then she stood still, remembering all the work that
she had been bidden to do and wondering what to begin first.
But as she looked she rubbed her eyes, for the yard was already neatly cleaned and the floors were nicely swept, and the
little doll was sitting in the storehouse picking the last black
grains and wild peas out of the quarter-measure of wheat.

Vasilissa ran and took the little doll in her arms. 'My dearest
little doll!' she cried. 'Thou hast saved me from my trouble!
Now I have only to cook the Baba Yaga's supper, since all the
rest of the tasks are done!'

'Cook it, with God's help,' said the doll, 'and then rest, and
may the cooking of it make thee healthy!' And so saying it
crept into her pocket and became again only a little wooden
doll.

So Vasilissa rested all day and was refreshed; and when it
grew toward evening she laid the table for the old witch's supper, and sat looking out of the window, waiting for her coming.
After a while she heard the sound of a horse's hoofs and the
man in black, on the coal-black horse, galloped up to the wall
gate and disappeared like a great dark shadow, and instantly it

became quite dark and the eyes of all the skulls began to glitter and shine.

Then all at once the trees of the forest began to creak and groan and the leaves and the bushes to moan and sigh, and the Baba Yaga came riding out of the dark wood in the huge iron mortar, driving with the pestle and sweeping out the trail behind her with the kitchen broom. Vasilissa let her in; and the witch, smelling all around her, asked, 'Well, hast thou done perfectly all the tasks I gave thee to do, or am I to eat thee for my supper?'

'Be so good as to look for thyself, grandmother,' answered Vasilissa.

The Baba Yaga went all about the place, tapping with her iron pestle, and carefully examining everything. But so well had the little doll done its work that, try as hard as she might, she could not find anything to complain of. There was not a weed left in the yard, nor a speck of dust on the floors, nor a single black grain or wild pea in the wheat.

The old witch was greatly angered, but was obliged to pretend to be pleased. 'Well,' she said, 'thou hast done all well.' Then, clapping her hands, she shouted, 'Ho! My faithful servants! Friends of my heart! Haste and grind my wheat!' Immediately three pairs of hands appeared, seized the wheat and carried it away.

The Baba Yaga sat down to supper, and Vasilissa put before her all the food from the oven, with kvass, honey, and red wine. The old witch ate it, bones and all, almost to the last morsel, enough for four strong men, and then, growing drowsy, stretched her bony legs on the stove and said, 'Tomorrow do as thou hast done today, and besides these tasks take from my storehouse a half-measure of poppy seeds and clean them one by one. Someone has mixed earth with them to do me a mischief and to anger me, and I will have them made perfectly clean.' So saying she turned to the wall and soon began to snore.

When she was fast asleep Vasilissa went into the corner, took the little doll from her pocket, set before it a part of the food that was left and asked its advice. And the doll, when it had eaten a little food and sipped a little drink, said, 'Don't

worry, beautiful Vasilissa! Be comforted. Do as thou didst
last night, say thy prayers and go to sleep.' So Vasilissa was
comforted. She said her prayers and went to sleep and did not
wake till next morning when she heard the old witch in the
yard whistling. She ran to the window just in time to see her
take her place in the big iron mortar, and as she did so the man
dressed all in red, riding on the blood-red horse, leaped over
the wall and was gone, just as the sun rose over the wild forest.

As it had happened on the first morning, so it happened now.
When Vasilissa looked she found that the little doll had finished
all the tasks excepting the cooking of the supper. The yard was
swept and in order, the floors were as clean as new wood, and
there was not a grain of earth left in the half-measure of poppy
seeds. She rested and refreshed herself till the afternoon, when
she cooked the supper, and when evening came she laid the
table and sat down to wait for the old witch's coming.

Soon the man in black, on the coal-black horse, galloped up
to the gate, and the dark fell and the eyes of the skulls began to
shine like day; then the ground began to quake, and the trees
of the forest began to creak and the dry leaves to rustle, and
the Baba Yaga came riding in her iron mortar, driving with her
pestle and sweeping away her path with her broom.

When she came in she smelled around her and went all
about the hut, tapping with the pestle; but pry and examine as
she might, again she could see no reason to find fault and was
angrier than ever. She clapped her hands and shouted, 'Ho! My
trusty servants! Friends of my soul! Haste and press the oil out
of my poppy seeds!' And instantly the three pairs of hands appeared, seized the measure of poppy seeds and carried it away.

Presently the old witch sat down to supper and Vasilissa
brought all she had cooked, enough for five grown men, and
set it before her, and brought beer and honey, and then she
herself stood silently waiting. The Baba Yaga ate and drank
it all, every morsel, leaving not so much as a crumb of bread;
then she said snappishly, 'Well, why dost thou say nothing, but
stand there as if thou wast dumb?'

'I spoke not,' Vasilissa answered, 'because I dared not. But
if thou wilt allow me, grandmother, I wish to ask thee some
questions.'

'Well,' said the old witch, 'only remember that every question does not lead to good. If thou knowest overmuch, thou wilt grow old too soon. What wilt thou ask?'

'I would ask thee,' said Vasilissa, 'of the men on horseback. When I came to thy hut, a rider passed me. He was dressed all in white and he rode a milk-white horse. Who was he?'

'That was my white, bright day,' answered the Baba Yaga angrily. 'He is a servant of mine, but he cannot hurt thee. Ask me more.'

'Afterwards,' said Vasilissa, 'a second rider overtook me. He was dressed in red and the horse he rode was blood-red. Who was he?'

'That was my servant, the round, red sun,' answered the Baba Yaga, 'and he, too, cannot injure thee,' and she ground her teeth. 'Ask me more.'

'A third rider,' said Vasilissa, 'came galloping up to the gate. He was black, his clothes were black and the horse was coal-black. Who was he?'

'That was my servant, the black, dark night,' answered the old witch furiously; 'but he also cannot harm thee. Ask me more.'

But Vasilissa, remembering what the Baba Yaga had said, that not every question led to good, was silent.

'Ask me more!' cried the old witch. 'Why dost thou not ask me more? Ask me of the three pairs of hands that serve me!'

But Vasilissa saw how she snarled at her and she answered, 'The three questions are enough for me. As thou hast said, grandmother, I would not, through knowing overmuch, become too soon old.'

'It is well for thee,' said the Baba Yaga, 'that thou didst not ask of them, but only of what thou didst see outside of this hut. Hadst thou asked of them, my servants, the three pairs of hands would have seized thee also, as they did the wheat and poppy seeds, to be my food. Now I would ask a question in my turn: How is it that thou hast been able, in a little time, to do perfectly all the tasks I gave thee? Tell me!'

Vasilissa was so frightened to see how the old witch ground her teeth that she almost told her of the little doll; but she bethought herself just in time, and answered, 'The blessing of my dead mother helps me.'

Then the Baba Yaga sprang up in a fury. 'Get thee out of my house this moment!' she shrieked. 'I want no one who bears a blessing to cross my threshold! Get thee gone!'

Vasilissa ran to the yard, and behind her she heard the old witch shouting to the locks and the gate. The locks opened, the gate swung wide, and she ran out onto the lawn. The Baba Yaga seized from the wall one of the skulls with burning eyes and flung it after her. 'There,' she howled, 'is the fire for thy stepmother's daughters. Take it. That is what they sent thee for, and may they have joy of it!'

Vasilissa put the skull on the end of a stick and darted away through the forest, running as fast as she could, finding her path by the skull's glowing eyes which went out only when morning came. Whether she ran a long way or a short way, and whether the road was smooth or rough, towards evening of the next day, when the eyes in the skull were beginning to glimmer, she came out of the dark, wild forest to her stepmother's house.

When she came near to the gate, she thought, 'Surely, by this time they will have found some fire,' and threw the skull into the hedge; but it spoke to her, and said, 'Do not throw me away, beautiful Vasilissa; bring me to thy stepmother.' So, looking at the house and seeing no spark of light in any of the windows, she took up the skull again and carried it with her.

Now since Vasilissa had gone, the stepmother and her two daughters had had neither fire nor light in all the house. When they struck flint and steel the tinder would not catch and the fire they brought from the neighbours would go out as soon as they carried it over the threshold, so that they had been unable to light or warm themselves or to cook food to eat. Therefore now, for the first time in her life, Vasilissa found herself welcomed. They opened the door to her and the merchant's wife was greatly rejoiced to find that the light in the skull did not go out as soon as it was brought in. 'Maybe the witch's fire will stay,' she said, and took the skull into the best room, set it on a candlestick and called her two daughters to admire it.

But the eyes of the skull suddenly began to glimmer and to glow like red coals, and wherever the three turned or ran the eyes followed them, growing larger and brighter till they

flamed like two furnaces, and hotter and hotter till the merchant's wife and her two wicked daughters caught fire and
were burned to ashes. Only Vasilissa the Beautiful was not
touched.

From Russian Wonder Tales *by Post Wheeler*

The Mother of the Self

The story of Vasilissa confronts us with the twin themes of the death of
her mother and the 'birth' of her doll. That the two coincide is the story's
way of telling us that one is the pre-requisite for the other. The death of
the mother is inevitably linked to the reception of the doll.

Obviously the 'mother' of the story is not the actual mother: children
receive dolls without their mother having to die first. The mother here is
the child's own origin, her true self, her innermost soul and spiritual part
that cannot fully enter this world and is therefore left in another. Every
childhood is the slow dying to this depth-dimension of soul. Every child
leaves the greater part of herself, her 'mother,' behind. This 'mother'
dies, or rather withdraws, and guides the child from another realm. But
a memory of her remains and that is the doll. She is all that is left of the
once-speaking animate world.

The story of Vasilissa links the protective powers of the higher self to
its representative: the doll. The doll conveys her mother's blessing to her,
consoles her and helps her in her need.

All dolls do that. To the child they stand as a memory of who they
truly are; they are the keeper of the child's initial intents, their wishes
and intentions before birth.

The doll is a little remnant of paradise, a picture of the higher self.
This is what makes Vasilissa's doll so *'very precious for there is no
other like it in the world.'* This is the true doll behind all dolls, of which
it makes sense to say: *'Carry it always about with thee in a pocket and
never show it to anyone.'* The true doll is always an invisible companion
and the outer doll its representative.

Outer dolls are little idols in the early years of matrilineal society and
demi-gods in the religion of childhood. They are worshipped with much
attention and surrounded with rituals by the child. This symbolic status
makes them more loved and cared for than other toys. They are the true
soulmates.

Rightly understood, the doll is the first real responsibility in the life of the child. It is the soul's own child, the first being that is totally entrusted to the child's care. To be given a doll is a deeply symbolic act, an act that means no less than: 'This is your first of tasks, the most important of all responsibilities, the care for your soul-child, your essential self.'

The reception of the doll is a ritual act, a symbolic teaching in a language the child can understand. The Persian poet, Rumi, eloquently expressed this in a parable.

> The master said there is one thing in this world which must never be forgotten. If you were to forget everything else, but are not to forget this, there would be no cause to worry, while if you remembered, performed and attended to everything else, but forgot that one thing, you would in fact have done nothing whatsoever. It is as if a king had sent you to a country to carry out one special, specific task. You go to the country and you perform a hundred other tasks, but if you have not performed the task you were sent for, it is as if you have performed nothing at all. So man has come into the world for a particular task, and that is his purpose. If he doesn't perform it, he will have done nothing.

The doll is the link to this foremost of responsibilities, to the task that we should never forget. Through caring for the doll the child begins to care for its higher self and its own mission in the world. Part of this care is the ritual feeding of the doll. Like Vasilissa, many children give their doll food to eat. They bestow reality on it and treat it like a real being.

The kvas and the breadcrumbs make her doll come alive. The sole diet of the higher self as well as that of every doll is love and attention. It is attention that keeps a doll alive. They rarely die of wear and tear as they can be patched *ad infinitum*. They die for lack of attention, when they are forgotten, ignored, or buried in a drawer. They have, however, remarkable powers of recovery and can quickly be resurrected from the dead.

The self is just like that. It thrives on attention and is diminished through lack of love. Forgotten it dies. Remembered it comes to life again.

Vasilissa is lucky in this respect. Her life forces her to keep constant communion with her doll. Every day she takes the doll from her pocket and feeds her kvas and bread. And every night the doll helps her. Left to her own devices she could not accomplish her many tasks. But what is impossible for her is well within the reach of her doll.

Life is just like that. Challenge after challenge comes our way: problems that cannot be solved, knots that can't be untied and questions that cannot be answered. We are helpless in the vicious circle of our insecurities, stranded on the rocks of reality. The severity of our trials, like Vasilissa's, increases during life. In Baba Yaga's hut they reach their terrifying peak.

Like all great tales, Vasilissa the Beautiful simultaneously tells the journey of the individual soul and that of humanity, the latter apparent in her meeting with the white, the red and the black rider, and eventually the fourth and most ghostly of them all, Baba Yaga, mounted on her mortar and pestle. Here the story parallels the four riders of the apocalypse from the book of Revelation. The first three are very similar, while Baba Yaga is an older, matriarchal version of the fourth and, like him, surrounded by the accoutrements of death. Bones and skulls are her home. This is the dead end of it all, the valley of shadows, the stove full of ash; the final place where souls are crushed by the mortar and pestle of time and held in a prison with locks like jawbones and sharp teeth barring the way. A place where everyone trembles like Vasilissa, and no one can escape.

Vasilissa is every one of us and the whole of humanity. She is the human soul that has come to meet the bare bones of the world, the place of skulls, the Golgotha of our time. Like her we all wrestle with death. We face environmental crises that seem insurmountable. Like her we hear the terrible noise, the trees that begin to groan, the branches that creak and the dry leaves that rustle at Baba Yaga's approach. Like Vasilissa we see a wall of bones made from every war that has swept the earth. Like her we watch the rich devour far more than their share while the poor are oppressed. And like her we come to get fire, to spark light from the flint of resistance. Our life is at stake, and our doll is our only hope — her presence alone preserves us from harm.

Vasilissa's tasks are, like ours, impossible to solve. Nobody can pick all the black grains from the quarter-measure of wheat or sort a half-measure of seeds in one night. These tasks are beyond human capacity and that is where they are solved. The doll — the higher self — sorts everything out.

The Material Doll

The story of Vasilissa invokes the very essence of the doll, its highest archetype. Dolls serve, of course, many more purposes. They are play-mates for the imagination of the child. They are friends populating chil-dren's homes and quiet family members on the fringe of adult life.

Ideally, dolls are made by a family member or friend, stitched with the care, love and attention of the maker. Such a doll is a real gift containing much of the giver. It is a tangible blessing bestowed in the beginning of life.

Vasilissa's doll looks just like herself. A true doll should look like the child. Not only that, it ought to mirror the child's moods. A true doll needs to be able to change its expression and even grow with the child. This may seem an impossible demand for the maker. And it is. It is one of those tasks that cannot be solved, like cleaning a half-measure of poppy seeds.

But having read Vasilissa you know what to do — leave the task to the doll. You do this by keeping the doll simple. Then she can easily master her complex task. See the doll below, made and sketched by Anne Williams. This is a doll for a young child. It is as simple as possible, free of all detail.

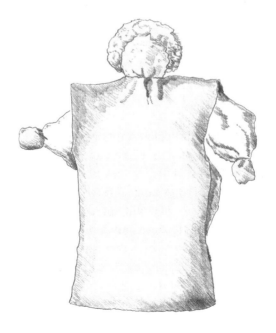

This doll has all faces because it has none. Bearing simply the outline of the human form, and unconstrained by any particular expression, it can express anything. This is a doll that can mirror all moods, that looks like the child when the child looks at it. A doll that can grow with the child, laugh and weep with the child. This is the magical doll that can be anything at any time, that comes to life when you attend to it, that solves all problems: one good night's sleep and in the morning problems are gone. This doll is easy to make. Its simplicity keeps it close to the mobility of the archetype.

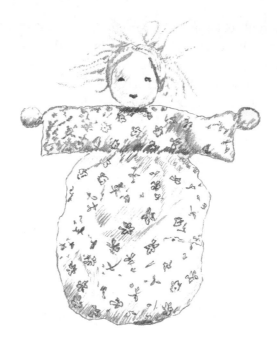

The doll above is more articulate in its expression. Mouth and eyes are clearly indicated. The hair is elaborate and the dress beautifully-shaped and patterned. This doll has moved away from the archetype but still retains the mobility to shape-shift with the child's imagination. A child beyond three years of age will appreciate the added details and the finery of dress. The eyes that are only hinted at allow a maximum of expression. These are the kind of eyes that can shine like fireflies or like glow-worms, like stars or like candles. The kind of eyes that Vasilissa's doll had — the kind that can shine for the child.

Dolls are indispensable in the kingdom of childhood. They are the kings and queens of this golden age. Among their courtiers are the animals and soft toys that populate the provinces of the child's soul: the much loved bears and seals, horses and striped tigers, dogs of every breed and cats of every kind of fur. This is the time for milk-white lambs and pigs of rosy complexion. Children love their felted zoo. This menagerie of soft toys is part of their imaginary sphinx, a memory of a long-lost time that is temporarily regained in these early years. Like the doll, these animals need to be simple rather than realistic, archetypal rather than naturalistic. Details are best left to the imagination, which will actively complete what is left unfinished. In this way children become co-creators in the reality of their fabulous world. They learn to approach the realm of the archetype through the life of the imagination.

So let your children enjoy the echoes of animism in our inanimate world. Allow them to revel in a paradise of their own making and the company of talking beasts. (Dinosaurs, by the way, were not among the original inhabitants of Paradise; nor were they carried aboard Noah's Ark. Their ecological niche is the dragon's cave we meet in later tales.)

The Re-enchantment of the World

Dolls stand for the self. Animals portray aspects of soul: they assist the soul in the assembling of its own world. Allow your child to be the Noah in the Ark of her inner life, a collector of talking beasts before the heavy rain of reason drowns her fragile world. In the meantime let them be part of your stories: like the dolls, they have much to tell.

The doll provides the best means for you to begin your story-making. Let her teach you. She is willing to help if you are willing to feed her. All she needs is your full attention. If you treat her with the respect she deserves she will come to life and tell *you* the very stories you need for your child. The stories she will want to tell first will be tailored to the young child, that speak in a language the child understands: the vernacular of the young soul; the forgotten language of paradise in which all things speak. The first creature to speak, of course, is the doll herself. Like all of us, she has her stories, and these are often unexpectedly helpful to the parent.

Here the doll is talking in a story by Mags Webster:

> I was asking the owl who sits on the tree outside our window,
> how can he see in the dark? And he told me that the stars and

the moon help him to see, and he even looks through the window and watches us asleep each night.

You may have noticed that dolls have a certain trait: they disappear for
times and then are suddenly back again. They walk in and out of our
attention. You may have wondered what they do during their absence.
It is in these times that they often have the most remarkable adventures.
And just as in Nandi Chinna's story, they like to talk about them when
they return to their family:

> Guess where I have been?
> I've been up in the air on the back of a bird.
> I was inside the blue sky.
> A bee flew past and buzzed in my ear.
> Then the bird flew down
> and gently put me
> right back here.

Children love to listen to the secret adventures of their doll. For the storyteller, the doll's encounters open the gates to the world where animals
talk and inanimate objects have own stories to tell.

In this world everything comes alive. Even the objects of modern
technology arise from their functional graves. The phone, the washing
machine and the vacuum cleaner belong to Baba Yaga's hut, the skull
and bones of our times. They are the rarely-acknowledged household
slaves that have fallen farthest from paradise. They represent the dead
end of nature, but they can be redeemed.

To the doll, as you have seen, nothing is impossible. She can successfully carry out the hardest tasks and can easily bestow personality
on electrical pets such as vacuum cleaners and fridges. Through her
guidance your old fridge turns into a trusty friend, toasters find excuses
for burning the toast and a temperamental frying pan won't stop talking.
Even the white goods in the laundry have something to say, as in this
story by Gaye O'Donnell:

> Sally the doll sat in the laundry leaning against the sink tap.
> 'Don't you ever get dizzy?' she asked. 'Not really,' said the
> dryer in a grumbling voice. 'Just a little hot and bothered.'
>   'Where does all the fluff come from?' asked Sally. 'Off the

clothes of course,' said the dryer with a giggle.

Sally heard a thump, strangely recurring. 'Ohhhhhh,' said the dryer with a groan, 'I wish she wouldn't do the sneakers, they give me such a bellyache.'

'There, there,' said Sally, patting the side of the dryer. 'Winter's nearly over.'

Through such stories the doll initiates the storyteller into a forgotten part of herself. She parts the hedges that have grown over the castle of childhood and awakens everything from the sleep of forgetting. The doll enlivens the world and returns things to beings that have a story to tell.

19. Taming Place and Time

The Homecoming

The mother is the first of homes for the child, the one from which all else unfolds. The body is next. Family and friends, the house, the garden, and nearby surroundings are other and increasingly more spacious homes.

Each child is a natural home-builder. The early years are given entirely to the activity of shaping the inherited body. It is like building an instrument to the requirements of a future musician. The eyes and the ears and the brain have to be tuned and the limbs and organs fashioned for the unique symphony of a life. This takes time and progresses in distinct stages.

Children map these stages through their drawings. The closed circle indicates a first kind of home found within. Later the motif of the house occurs in many variations. The making of cubbies and hideouts may be seen as an expression of yearning for home. Children often daydream about their own place, a cubby (den) or tree house. Such dreams can be clearly remembered in adult life, as in the case of Jesse Williamson:

> There was once a little boy called Jamey, who lived by the tall
> cliffs that rose out of the sea. Jamey loved it when the storms
> came and a chill wind would rush in off the ocean. He loved to
> stand on the solid rocks and taste the salty ocean spray that the
> wind brought him. And if the wind blew too hard he would go
> inside a little house that was nestled up to the cliffs and tucked
> in away under them. He would shut the strong wooden door
> and keep out the wind. The cottage had thick snuggly curtains
> which he would draw so that then the house was lit only by
> the soft glow of an open fire. In front of the fire was a soft rug
> where he would sit to warm his cold feet and wiggling toes.

This story transports me back to my own childhood. My picture of my ideal cubby home was very different, but the feeling was exactly the same.

Recalling our own feelings is a good preparation for telling a story. It helps us find the emotional perspective and the right tone. It prepares the appropriate mood, the womb out of which stories are born.

You can help your child find his way home through a story that makes houses into homes, back yards into gardens and sandpits into castles. I call this story the Homecoming. It is the kind of story that transforms the foreign into the familiar and turns every suburban labyrinth into a meaningful place.

In all cases of geographical bewilderment, naming through story assists the taming of place. It paves the winding road all the way home to the body. This story centres the soul and prepares for it a place to feel safe.

All you need for the Homecoming story is to invent a hero by means of a name and then describe the hero's home, which will resemble the home of your child. Start at the periphery of your child's experience and spiral inwards. It will add to the story if you begin it with a magical phrase such as: 'In a land far away ...' or 'A long, long time ago ...'

Here is an example by Ute ten Hompel:

> Once upon a time there was a little girl whose name was Lucy.
> She lived high up in the mountains in a house made of wood.
> Even the roof was covered with wooden shingles. It had a big
> chimney and windows with a cross. Lucy's room was behind
> the front door. Her door was out of the same wood as her big
> bed that was covered with white linen. In front, stood a shelf
> with her two dolls, some beautiful crystals, and a basket full
> of dried flowers and sea shells. On the floor lay a rug, soft and
> warm. The cupboard stood in the corner and in it were all her
> clothes and clothes for her doll.

In the imaginal world of childhood the home represents the body. Homecoming stories assist the child's homecoming into the body and layer the child's surroundings like a protective onion-skin around its soul. They provide a buffer of meaning and a narrative form of orientation.

Starting with the greater picture such as house or garden, or the immediate surrounds, proceed slowly inwards. End in the child's room or special corner and bring in all the particulars that populate its realm, and remember that inanimate objects are still alive for the child. The story below by Grace McQuade does all this and enlarges the theme by encompassing the sojourn of a child's day:

> Once upon a time in a green land far away a little bird took
> to the sky and flew and flew and flew over the sea till it saw a
> wide brown land with houses on it. It flew to a house with a
> tin roof and smelled the roses growing near the red brick walls
> and settled on a white windowsill. The window was open and
> the blue curtains flapped in the gentle breeze. In the room was
> a bed with a blue quilt over it. By the bed was a chest of draw-
> ers on which there were some soft toys. A yellow bear, a red
> and blue turtle and a green frog. On a small table by the bed
> was a little red train. The door of the room had a name on it:
> Luke.
>   The boy was there now, asleep in his bed. The bird began
> its morning song. The boy opened his eyes and listened to the
> bird's song. Then he jumped out of bed to play. He played
> all day with the little red train, the yellow bear, the red and
> blue turtle and the green frog. Then he was tired and ready to
> lie down in the bed, under the blue quilt in the room with his
> name on the door. But where was the little bird who had sung
> on the white windowsill with the blue curtains flapping? It had
> gone now, past the red brick walls and the roses with their per-
> fume, away over the tin roof, up into the sky where the houses
> looked small and away over the sea, flying, flying, flying till
> it came to the green land and perched on a branch of a large
> leafy tree where it put its head in its feathers and slept too.

A story like this increases the sense of place through the double dose of naming. Once the child has begun to develop his own imagination at the age of four or five, you may add more touches of your own imagination to make the story more interesting. Mags Webster has done this in the story below:

> Once upon a time there was a little girl called Mary and she
> lived in a village on the edge of a huge forest, and Mary's
> home was the very last cottage on the very last street on the

very edge of the village before you got to the forest. Beside
Mary's home was the tallest pine tree you've ever seen, and in
the tree, way up in the branches, there lived an owl. And the owl
was friends with Mary and she would swoop down each night
to the lowest branch in the tallest tree to tap on the window pane
of Mary's bedroom. And Mary would be tucked up tight in her
bed, as cosy as anything under her grandmother's patchwork
quilt. And Mary would say goodnight to the owl, and give her
a wave before turning over and snuggling down under the quilt,
which was made of patches all the colours of the rainbow, with
stripes and spots and flowers. And somewhere in the middle of
the quilt there was a patch that wasn't like any of the others. It
was a very special patch. It was a magic patch, and the threads
holding it in place were strands of fairy hair. And if Mary
touched this patch, she turned into a little firefly and she could
fly to the window and out to her friend the owl, and perch beside
her on the lowest branch of the tallest tree.

Another way to approach this story is to follow the example of the old
children's verse 'The Key to the Kingdom,' and let your tale spiral in and
out of your child's reality. Nandi Chinna has done this in her tale:

On a hill above the ocean is a big brick house
On the roof of the house sit ten grey pigeons
In the garden of the house green grass grows
Amongst the green grass scratch three brown hens
In the kitchen of the house is a red table and around the red
    table are four red chairs
On the red table is a wooden bowl
Inside the wooden bowl are twelve ripe plums
On one red chair sits a small boy with sticky red plum juice all
    over his face
All over his face is sticky red plum juice
In a wooden bowl on the red table are eleven ripe plums
On the red table in the kitchen
In the big brick house.

This story intensifies the sense of place by spiralling in and out of the
child's reality. Spiralling in with story helps the child to take hold of its

home and body. Spiralling out may assist the transition into the world of dreams, as Julie Dickinson illustrates:

> It was Saturday and Emmie Lou's mother had taken her to her first ballet lesson and Emmie Lou was very excited. That night she could not go to sleep so she slipped out of bed and tried on her new pink ballet shoes and laced the ties, criss-cross up her legs. She pointed her toe as Miss Penelope had taught her and suddenly she was off!
>
> She danced down the stairs tippety tap, across the soft green grass swishety swish, over the white picket fence ploppity plop, and then she leapt into the air, whirling and whizzing, pirouetting and spiralling up to the top of a fir tree in the square of the neighbouring village. Standing on one toe she gazed in delight over the sleeping village and the surrounding forest and felt very close to the stars twinkling above her.
>
> Suddenly the village clock struck twelve and a cloud passed over the moon. A shudder ran through Emmie Lou and her toes twitched inside her pink ballet shoes, and in a trice she started pirouetting and spiralling into the air, whirling and whizzing across the village, landing ploppity plop over the white picket fence. Then swishety swish over the soft green grass, and tippety tap up the stairs to her little blue room and flippety flop into her nice warm bed — still wearing her new pink ballet shoes with the laces criss-crossed up her legs.

Take care that the limits of the story do not exceed the geography of the child's soul-experience. A neighbouring village and the visible stars are part of the young child's immediate world, but the solar system, the earth and the continents are generally not. A child's interior map only includes what has actually been seen and experienced. If the sea is not a known experience, leave it out. Start where you are.

Initiation into Time

Young children have no concept of time. Tell them to wait five minutes or two hours or until tomorrow — it all means the same to them: not now. And since now is all they know, the reaction is usually intense.

Children have no relation to the staccato of fragmented time. They are still attuned to the slow and steady pendulum swing of their biological clock, with its occasional chiming of seasons and its clear ciphers of night and day, meal-time, rest-time, playtime.

Children need to be initiated into time. As adults we forget the terrors of untamed time, but imagine for a moment living in a house where the location of rooms and furniture and everything else is constantly changing, and you get a spatial inkling of the stress a child experiences in the chaos of untamed time.

Initiation into time takes many years and is best achieved through rituals of regularity. A child thrives on regularity. Regularity means security and security means happiness. A well-established morning routine saves us from inventing each morning anew — along with endless negotiation and unnecessary power struggles. Through routine, the child develops a lifelong alliance with time, and the ability to flow with rather than push against its mighty current. Though it takes time and effort to establish a routine, it saves time in the end. One such routine is the telling of stories such as the Adventurous Day.

The Adventurous Day

The story of the adventurous day helps to befriend Giant Time. It calms the avalanche of events and assists in digesting the chunks of daily experience. Told in the evening, it directs the chaotic currents of time into the riverbed of sleep.

The adventurous day is the simplest of stories, and an excellent place to start your career as storyteller. As in the last exercise, you begin by inventing a name for your imaginary hero, who will experience in story-space what your child has experienced during the day. Through this device the story becomes separated enough from the child's reality to be interesting.

Starting with an invocatory phrase like 'Once upon a time' increases the impact. Such words have a magical effect: they are doorways into the timeless realm of story.

Remember that the child's life *is* adventurous. Every back yard is a world to be explored, every outing a journey into the unknown. Every day is an adventure of its own. Take the child's world as seriously as you do your own. Treat it as story-worthy, and retell your child's day in a lively manner. There is no need to dramatize it. Just try to see the pictures inwardly, then elaborate on the particulars. Do not be afraid of repeating basic details, they will most likely be reassuring rather than boring.

A good time to start this story is at the age of three, when the child begins to say 'I.' Here is an example I have written to illustrate this:

> Once there was a girl called Mira who lived with her mum and a cat in a large house. The cat's name was Mr Pussum. Every morning when Mira woke up she looked for Mr Pussum. And sometimes Mr Pussum was there and sometimes he wasn't. This time he was already up and about. So Mira ran straight into the kitchen. And there was her mum and Mr Pussum.
>
> Mira gave Mr Pussum a bowl of milk and Mr Pussum licked it all clean. Then her mum gave Mira a bowl of porridge and Mira ate it all up.
>
> Then Mira took all her wooden blocks from her basket and began to build. First she made a tower that was almost as tall as she was, but the tower did not want to be so tall and fell down. And when the tower had once more fallen down all by itself and then once more because Mira wanted it to, Mira started to build a house for her doll Sheryl, with a garage on the side.
>
> Then it was time to go shopping. Mira and her mum passed the yellow Post Office at the corner of their street and the school with the flag on the flag-post waving hello to them. At the supermarket Mira climbed into a large shopping trolley and helped her mum to stack all the cans and packets.
>
> They drove home, past the flag on the flag-post waving goodbye to them and past the yellow Post Office at the corner of their street. Back home Mira's mother started to cook. Mira took some pots and started to cook too. Mira stirred and stirred and stirred and when she had stirred enough, lunch was ready. Her Mum gave Mira a bowl of soup and Mira was so hungry she ate it all. Then Mira wanted a toast with honey, but mum said that the honey always had a nap at noon and that she had to wait until afternoon tea.
>
> While her mum washed the dishes Mira gave Sheryl a bowl of the soup she had made. Sheryl was very hungry and ate it

all up. Then Sheryl wanted honey. But Mira said the honey was having a nap and she had to wait for afternoon tea. So Sheryl and Mira had a nap and afterwards Mira went to play in the sandpit. When the honey was awake again, Mira and Sheryl and Mum had their tea. Mr Pussum came and sniffed at the toast, but did not want honey. 'I prefer cat food,' he said and slinked away. Mira too had a lot to do and followed him into the yard.

Mira baked sand-cakes all afternoon, until her mother called her. She had found two lonely woodblocks complaining about being left behind. Mira quickly put them back and all the other blocks cheered as they returned to their home. Mira gave Mr Pussum his food, had a bath and then ate supper with her mum. She was very hungry from all that baking and cooking and shopping and building and bathing and ate everything on her plate.

Then it was time for bed. Mira said good night to Mr Pussum, took Sheryl and carefully tucked her under her sheet. Mum told Mira a story, sang a song and kissed her good night. When her mum closed the door to Mira's room, Mira's eyes closed too and she fell fast asleep.

The Pitfalls of Thought and Sentiment

There are two pitfalls that can spoil a hero's adventures. The first is thought. Heroes are doers, not thinkers. They get up and get on with it. They don't contemplate or plan ahead. They follow their feet. Children are such heroes. Avoid weighing down their actions with the heavy burden of thought like this:

> Lucy lay in bed for a while and thought, shall I go outside or shall I crawl into Mummy and Daddy's bed or shall I …

Even if the child is a bit ponderous, it need not be encouraged in story time. The story is not just about the child. It is about the hero.

The other trap is sentimentality. True heroes want no bar of it. All it does is drown their adventures in the syrup of misplaced feelings:

It was the most beautiful morning. George woke with a smile.
His mummy had prepared a yummy porridge and a cup of his
favourite drink, lovely milk with sweet honey.

Use words like beautiful, lovely and yummy sparingly, like spice on
good food. It goes without saying that mornings are beautiful, that the
parents are the best of parents, that the food is good and honey-sweet.

When George woke up he could smell the porridge his mother
had made. He got out of bed, brushed his teeth, washed his
face and ran into the kitchen …

That is a hero's way to wake up and tackle his day.
   Take your clues from good stories and fairytales. They have a tale to
tell and they do it. They don't linger in elaborate description and ornate
language, they march straight in to the adventure.

In the next story, Mags Webster adds a teddy to the adventures of Jack:

Today started very, very early, almost before the first birds
woke up, when Jack thought that Teddy had jumped out of
bed, because Teddy was lying on the floor. So Jack had to get
out of bed and pick Teddy up and take him into Mummy's
room to warm him up. Mummy said, 'Why don't you bring
Teddy downstairs, and he can help me make breakfast and sit
beside you while you drink your milk?' So that is just what
Jack did, and later on, Teddy watched while Mummy helped
Jack put on his clothes.
   Jack decided he wanted to go for a walk, so he and Mummy
and Teddy went outside into the sunshine and walked along
the path for ever such a long time, so that Jack could say hello
to all his favourite trees. By the time they got home, everyone
was hungry, even Teddy, so it was time for lunch. Mummy
decided to make some scrambled eggs, but she needed Jack
to help her whisk the eggs before they went into the sauce-
pan. Jack was very brave and stood on a chair to help, and he
whisked very hard, so hard that some of the egg flew out of the
bowl and landed on Teddy! But Teddy didn't mind.
   After lunch, it was time to play in the garden, so Jack and

Teddy sat on Jack's little tractor so they could be farmers. And everybody knows that farmers get very hungry, and very dirty, so when Jack and Teddy came back inside for tea, they had to wash all the mud off them, even from behind their ears, before they could eat anything. After that, Mummy said it was time for bed, because Jack had been so busy all day that Teddy was tired out!

And so up they went to bed, and Jack climbed all the stairs without stopping once. And now he's tucked up in bed with Teddy, but tonight, Teddy's sleeping on the other side of the bed, next to the wall, so that he'll be safe and sound and won't jump out of bed — until the morning.

To tell this story successfully you have to distinguish between the essential and the non-essential from a child's point of view. It helps to keep the hero active by emphasizing his part in the unfolding of the day. Stories are always selective of reality — they sift reality for what it's worth. They distil the events for whatever spirit they contain.

20. Coming to the Senses

Now that your child's soul is safely anchored in time and place, you can begin to lead her further by means of story. A secure way to do this is to elaborate on the child's experiences in the sense world. Use the hero to widen your child's horizon. If the child climbed a tree in the late afternoon, let your hero do the same. But let the hero make observations the child has not yet made. The hero sees, hears, touches, smells and senses more than the child.

Your hero may become aware of a bird nesting in the foliage or a caterpillar chewing its way through a fat green leaf. Describe in detail all that the hero experiences. Let your child see through the eyes of your story into the wonders of the world. Bring the bird to life in your words. Name it. If it was a blue wren describe the hero's delight in its intense blue colour, its quick movements and alert eyes. Your devotion to detail will remind the child of what she has already vaguely perceived and prepare her to observe more closely on the next occasion.

Keep the story within your child's horizon. Use your back yard or a nearby park rather than the African jungle. Avoid kangaroos if you live in New York and elephants if your home is the Australian bush. Celebrate what is at your doorstep and keep your tale anchored in the reality of the child. Nothing is ordinary to a child; everything is new and interesting. If it is not, make it so by means of your story.

Awe is a natural state of the child. Only in our 'unnatural' society is it so easily lost or dulled. story medicine will help to revive awe and offer an immediate means of environmental education through the sense of wonder.

Tales celebrating nature offer fresh encounters with the slow teachings of the garden snail and the work ethic of the earthworm. They alert the child to the two-way traffic of ants over a piece old bark and the birdsong in the morning air.

For the story-maker too this is an opportunity to undo the knots that familiarity has tied into your own soul, and look again with wonder at the revelations of this world. It is a chance of a second childhood and a return to a way of seeing you may have lost.

Avoid explanation in this kind of story. Do not burden the child with too much knowledge. Simply describe what is to be seen. Let the things and creatures and events speak for themselves. Elaborate on what can or could be observed in the tree, the back yard and the pond or on the way to a park as in this story by Nandi Chinna:

> Sproutie and Auntie went to the park. They packed a bag with hats and a water bottle and some bananas. Sproutie carried the bag on her back.
>
> They walked up the steep hill. Sproutie ran ahead of Auntie.
>
> Past the purple daisies.
>
> Past the sweet smelling Jasmine vine.
>
> Past the brick house with the green roof.
>
> Past the vacant block with the broken shopping trolley.
>
> Past the bus stop.
>
> To the big green grass of the park!
>
> Sproutie tore off her shoes and ran as fast as she could around and around on the soft green grass. Auntie tried to catch up but Sproutie was too fast.
>
> She ran to the playground. There was a sand pit with swings and slides and a whizzy-go-round. Sproutie ran to the slide. She looked up at the ladder. It was very high. She put one foot on the first rung. The metal was warm and smooth. She reached up for the next rung with her hands. Auntie watched and called, 'Go on Sproutie, you can do it.'
>
> Sproutie lifted up her other foot onto the next rung and Ho. She was up! Reaching her hands up one by one, feet, hands, feet, hands, soon her feet touched the top of the slide.
>
> She looked down. It was a long way. Auntie clapped and cheered.
>
> Sproutie laughed and laughed as she sat down at the top of the slide. She gave a push and with a 'whoosh' she was back down at the bottom again.

Like this, the story becomes a stimulus for the child's own observations. The purple daisies and the sweet jasmine vine will wait for Sproutie the next time she passes by. She will even notice the broken shopping trolley on the block before the bus stop and the warm rungs of the ladder in the playground.

The pictures you bring to the story are like seeds that will grow into reality. I imagine these stories acting on the child in much the way that cave paintings acted on humanity in prehistory, supporting our passage from dreamtime to reality. For that is what our story does. It supports the child's coming to terms with her environment. Here is an example by Suzanne Smith that combines observation and education:

> In the early light of the morning when the sun was still low in the sky and the shadows were on the trees so that they looked all black, Amber woke up and got out of bed. She put her slippers on and rubbed her eyes — everyone was still asleep. She was the only one awake and inside and outside it was very quiet.
>
> Amber walked out of her bedroom and went to the kitchen. She took the key to the back door off the low hook. She pushed a stool close to the door and climbed up on it. Then she undid the lock to the door and pushed it open. The light from the sky came into the room, but it was not bright light like in the day. The sun was still waking up, just like Amber, so the colours in the sky were orange and yellow and just a little bit of blue. Amber went outside; she crossed the threshold of the verandah and went out onto the grass. She heard a noise and looked up to see a big flock of birds way up in the sky, squawking and making a lot of noise. They flew up and away and over the house.
>
> Amber walked across the grass to the chicken coop. The chickens were just getting up too. She went to the fence and squatted down and watched them. They were walking around and pecking at the ground or at the feeder. Some of them were having a drink. One chicken was kicking the dirt with its feet and making dust go everywhere. Some of the chickens were still in the coop; she could hear them making noises. All of a sudden one chicken came over to where Amber was sitting.
>
> 'Bikerk! Hello Amber,' said the chicken.
>
> 'Hello,' said Amber.
>
> The chicken watched Amber very closely with one eye. Amber looked at the chicken and could see its eye, she looked at the feathers of the chicken, and they were brown and red. She

wanted to pat the chicken but could not fit her hand through the fence.

'Bikerk! Where is your mother?' said the chicken.

'They are still asleep, I am the only one awake,' said Amber.

The chicken said, 'Come with me and I will show you something.'

Amber walked around and the chicken showed her a hole in the fence. The chicken walked through the hole to the long grass, where Amber saw, hidden in the grass an egg. Amber crouched down and looked at the egg, she wanted to touch it, and she asked the chicken if it was all right to pick it up and the chicken said, 'Yes.' Amber picked up the egg, it was warm. She held it in her two hands and it made them warm up.

'The googy-egg is warm,' said Amber.

'Yes,' said the chicken, 'that is because it has just been laid. When it comes out of the chicken it is warm cause the chicken keeps it warm with her body.'

Amber thought about this for a long time. Then she reached out to touch the chicken on the feathers. Just as she did that, the chicken ran away.

'Come back chicken!' But the chicken ran away back through the hole and into the chicken coop and Amber was left holding the egg. She heard a noise and looked up and saw that the house had a light on in the kitchen. She went into the kitchen and held the egg up for her mother to see and as she held it up she smiled a big smile. Mum said, 'Wow,' and then she said, 'Would you like to have that egg for breakfast?'

Stories like this pre-digest the world. They continue to do what the mother does in the first years of life. By naming the world they make it a hospitable place. A story like this gently awakens the senses. It alerts the child to the fabric of qualities in which all life is wrapped and opens its mind to the poetry of everything.

Once you have the knack of this kind of story and your child's imagination has begun to stir you will be ready to make a new acquaintance, the 'imaginal ally' — the new hero of the stories you are going to tell.

21. Imaginal Allies

The imaginal ally is the hero that helps you tell your tale. It is indispensable for story-makers and gives you the confidence you need. Imaginal allies are a kind of invisible doll that whispers stories in your ear. And it is at this point that you can begin to approach them.

Imaginal allies are always helpful and as real as you will have them. They are entirely made of your attention. Visited frequently, they grow in size and acquire a life of their own. With a good education and proper care they become a source of unlimited support. Luckily, they are educated by the same stories you would tell your child, so you need not double up. They will grow on you, with you and through you, and sometimes even in spite of you.

Above all, imaginal allies are great storytellers. Their story is their mission, their only purpose in life. They have nothing else to do — they *are* their stories. They wait for ages for someone to hear their tale. They are always ready when you are. They are part of your own household of imaginary and invisible friends, soulmates and muses.

Finding and Naming the Ally

To begin with, I recommend modelling your imaginal ally on your child. You will start to swim in the shallows rather than in the depths. Once you have learned to stay afloat in the waters of the imagination you can venture further as you please. If you do not have a child, perhaps there is still a significant child in your life. If there is not, then let your imagination provide one.

A secure way to begin is by elaborating on the hero of your previous stories, the one who mirrors your child. All you need do now is take the hero a step further from your child to make him more interesting and the story more adventurous. Retain the parallels in the things that matter to the child and take creative licence with the rest. The similarities will make a powerful bond between the child and the hero–ally of your story. The differences will liberate the hero from the bounds of reality to adventure freely in the realm of the imagination.

Names have the power to invoke story. For the imaginal ally, names are their point of contact. Always invoke the name and use it frequently to charge the imagination. The longer the name the more substance it gives. An impressive name anchors the imaginal ally in the reality of sound and places him more firmly in the imagination. Think of Eustace Clarence Scrubb or the alliteration of Bastian Balthazar Bux.

Loosening the Reins

It may help to create your ally in two steps. Take your starting point from the actual description of your child and then add fiction, sparingly at first. Let the hero grow in parallel with the child's imagination and your capability as a story-maker. Nandi Chinna's Sproutie Greensmith illustrates both steps of this process. In the first, the description is gleaned from reality:

> Sproutie Greensmith has short blonde wispy hair that sticks up
> from the top of her head like a spike. She is short with a round
> rosy face and almond shaped green eyes. She does not wear
> shoes and she can run very fast. She wears dark green overalls.
> She is five years old. She lives at the end of the street where
> the white cedar grows, in a house with a green tiled roof.

The second step is to add imaginal detail. This is done by loosening some of the reins and tying them to the imagination. The imaginal hero needs appropriate clothes and proper equipment for the tasks ahead. He may or may not be older than the child, but his new features clearly distinguish him as a native of the imagination.

Describe your imaginal ally as clearly as possible. The more detail you can muster the more firmly he will take root in your imagination — and your child's. Your ally will repay your attention to personal detail with the detailed accounts of his stories. Your tale will inevitably become more artistic and its content more interesting to the child. This kind of story comes into play when the child's own imagination emerges.

Here is Nandi Chinna's description of her imaginal ally, based on Sproutie Greensmith:

> Sproutie Greensmith has short blonde wispy hair that sticks up
> from the top of her head like a spike. She is short with a round

rosy face and almond shaped green eyes. She does not wear
shoes and she can run very fast. She wears dark green overalls.
She is five years old.

Sproutie Greensmith lives at the edge of a city where the
red river gums tower above the rooftops and the back yards are
bursting with choko vines and plum trees.

Sproutie has a red bicycle called Merida that she keeps in
her bedroom. Whenever she needs to go somewhere she sits
in the saddle and whispers, 'Merida take me to the beach,'
or 'Merida take me to the park,' and Merida zooms off down
streets and around corners until they reach their destination.

In Merida's basket is a special bunch of flowers. Whenever Sproutie is hungry she sniffs the flowers and thinks of a
favourite food, and on each stalk in place of a flower, appears a
banana, an ice cream, or a honey sandwich.

Every night before she goes to sleep Sproutie puts a rug
over Merida and says, 'Goodnight Merida, see you in the
morning.'

The earlier story forms a rung on the ladder of the imagination. Do not
hesitate to repeat details. Children love repetition and gain joy from prior
acquaintance with stories. They meet them like an old friend.

Imaginal Adventuring

The imagination is born in stages. Before the age of three the child
is too closely woven into the mother's soul to develop his own life of
fancy. The forces of fantasy are active in the body, and when they have
done their work there they are gradually liberated into the life of the
imagination. Energy that went into the body now unfolds into the life
of fantasy.

In the first stage the child is inspired by whatever comes his way. His
imagination begins to add to reality what reality lacks. A stick can be
tree or a house or a door, a chair can be a castle or a car, a train or a truck.
Your imagination does the same when you add fiction to fact to your
stories. In this way your process as storyteller parallels the process of the
child. Your story will enhance your own imagination as well as that of
your child, and each will be strengthened by the other's company.

To begin, let your imaginal ally take the lead in adventures that highlight your child's day. Let him take some incident a step further into adventure. If your child has climbed only a little way up the tree, let the ally disappear into its topmost foliage. You will most likely be giving back to the child what your adult perception has taken away. Use the techniques introduced in previous chapters as Erica Bonsall has done in this story:

> Shilo Brannigan awoke to the sounds of the willie wagtail outside his window. 'Cha-cha-cha, cha-cha-cha,' the willie wagtail sounded cross. Shilo leapt out of bed and ran outside, stopping only to slip his boots onto bare feet. The boots were scratchy but Shilo didn't notice. He ran to the tall white gum tree with its patches of dark brown, and his boots crunched on the dried up leaves beneath. He looked into the tree to see the willie wagtail. She was sitting on her small cup-like mud-nest, her tail wagging furiously, her wings flapping as she darted at the tawny frogmouth which sat coolly on the same branch a little further along.
>
> Small muted sounds came from the nest and Shilo knew that the babies he could not see were still there. Without hesitating, Shilo ran to the shed and dragged the old wooden ladder through the grass and dried up leaves. He struggled to set the ladder up beneath the tree and began to climb it. The willie wagtail was angry and did not notice him; the tawny frogmouth sat quite still, eyeing the nest and the baby birds, waiting patiently; watching.
>
> As Shilo came to the top of the ladder he reached out to steady himself and the movement caused the tawny frogmouth to look at him. Shilo caught his breath then flapped his arms at the startled frogmouth for all he was worth, and with what looked to be a careless shrug, the large bird flew away. The wagtail flew to Shilo's arm. 'Thank you,' the mother said, relieved, and flew back to her babies where she fussed and chatted, soothing them. Shilo dragged the ladder back to the shed and went inside for breakfast.

Once you are comfortable writing stories that did not happen but could have, you can take the next step. Your imagination will be ready and so will the child's.

Allow the hero to go further than your child would ever go. This does not mean you should rush him into adventures that he is not ready to face and you are not ready to tell. Proceed slowly. Follow the example of children who experiment with their boundaries. To begin with, they are always cautious. They take a step and immediately return.

Do the same with your ally and your imagination. Observe children in their play and elaborate on the clues their own imagination provides. In the story below Suzanne Smith has delicately interwoven play and imagination:

> Amber and Georgie went to play behind the sheds. They walked through the grass that was long and yellow. Behind the sheds was an old car. It had no doors or windows and the seats were very dusty and covered in spider webs.
>
> 'Wanna go for a drive?' said Amber. 'Yes,' said Georgie, and they jumped inside the car, dusted off the old cobwebs and sat down on the brown seats.
>
> Amber started to make the steering wheel turn but she couldn't see where she was going. So she stood up on the seat and Georgie stood up too.
>
> 'Start the car,' said Georgie.
>
> 'Okay,' said Amber. She pretended to turn the key and heard the engine revving up.
>
> 'Let's go!' she said, and they did.
>
> They passed Bluey the old dog, asleep in her kennel.
>
> They drove around the sheds and past the tractor and all the tools. Next they went past the shearing shed. It was empty but they could still smell all the wool that had once been in there.
>
> They saw sheep on the side of the road.
>
> Amber said that she could see a puddle in the middle of the road, up ahead. But when they got up close it had disappeared. Georgie said that it was called a mirage, but Amber still didn't know where all the water had gone.
>
> They drove and drove. Amber held the steering wheel and spun it around. She looked at the car. It was all brown where the paint had peeled off. She pulled on the seat belts. Georgie played with the radio. She started singing, 'Clap clap clap if you feel you want to … ooooh, oooooh.' And they did clap.
>
> They drove a long way from home that day.

They drove and drove. They drove into town and did some shopping and Georgie went to see a man about a dog.

Then they got into the car and drove back to the farm. They made the steering wheel go around and jumped on the seats. They saw sheep and cows. They waved to people in other cars. They turned into the front drive, past the dam, past the shearing sheds, past Bluey dog sleeping in her kennel, past the tractor and all the tools, and pretty soon they were back in the long yellow grass behind the sheds.

They stopped the car and Amber turned off the key. They were home.

This form of story is a good place to use your immediate surroundings for humorous incidents, exciting adventures and convoluted tales.

Good humour, by the way, is almost always appropriate and stimulates both the teller and the tale. How to use humour therapeutically is the theme of a later chapter, but you need not wait for that. You can apply it with great benefit in the stories you are telling now. Humour is a true panacea and an indispensable ingredient in story medicine.

Walking on Water

Reality is the solid ground beneath our feet. It offers consistent support. The realm of the imagined is less concrete. It lacks definition and clear outlines and is never static; it changes continuously. It is alive and has no other limits than those we bestow on it. In this world everything is possible and nothing is out of our reach.

But the very strength of the imaginal is also its weakness. We must, therefore, negotiate our entry into this world carefully. The story we are about to tell will help us to enter this new realm in safety. It will help us to find our way through the labyrinth of possibilities and traverse the landscape of the imagination. It will teach us how to 'walk on water.'

We have already begun by letting go of the reins and allowing the imaginative ally to transgress the laws of this world. In the beginning it may be advantageous to have some idea of how far you want your ally to venture, but do not rigidly impose this as a limit, or plan the adventures in detail. Think of it as a suggestion and watch to see what your hero makes of it. You can sit back and watch your ally perform. Just observe and then describe what you see.

If you are a beginner this takes some trust. It takes faith in your ally, the same faith it takes to walk on water. It may need practice. You may find your faith holds you up for a short while, only to sink into the plot-less abyss with no idea where to go. This tends to happen when you become conscious of yourself, rather than remaining present and aware with your ally. At moments of hesitation you lose trust in your ally and that is when you sink. You can expect this to happen in the beginning, so it is advisable to practise in the shallows. If it still feels too daunting, use a puddle. Start with the smallest part of imagination supported by a large part of reality and take if from there.

You will find support in all that you have acquired in the previous chapters. Use the power of naming. Ground your story in local reality and elaborate on the details. Set it in the past. Take the journey through the senses to gain momentum. And if you still find yourself starving for lack of story, remember the richness of the animated world.

Here is a story by Jean Hudson involving a mermaid to whet your adventurous spirit:

> Lucinda Jane lay on the bow of her father's fishing boat, gaz-ing into the cerulean water, its surface smooth as glass. The lull of the ocean made her drowsy. Through heavy eyelids, she saw in the water below her a mermaid. Blonde hair flowed about her, and she wore a necklace of pearls and shells.
>
> Lucinda Jane slipped into the water and took the mermaid's outstretched hand. They dived deep into the ocean through shafts of light with dolphins swimming beside them. Nep-tune's garden glowed with pink and purple coral. Beneath swaying seaweed they found a treasure chest overflowing with precious jewels. The mermaid placed a tiny pearl in Lucinda Jane's hand. Lucinda Jane put it in the front pocket of her jeans. Silver fish guided them back to the boat.
>
> Lucinda Jane opened her eyes, she still lay on the bow of the boat — but her clothes were dry. She looked deep into the water and waved farewell to the mermaid.
>
> 'Did you have a nice sleep?' asked her father.
>
> 'Actually, I was swimming with a mermaid.'
>
> She reached into her pocket. The tiny pearl felt warm in her hand.

Invocation and Silence

The step from reality into actual imagination can be a challenge. If you do not find it easy yet to walk on the water of your imagination, you can help yourself with the invocation of story.

The invocation does to a story what a name does to the hero. It calls it into being and brings it into story reality. Invocations like 'Once upon a time,' or 'In olden times when wishing still helped,' never fail to transport us into story place and time. They are door openers into the imagination, like an overture that sets the mood before the curtain is raised.

Invocations can help to put stories on the pedestal of the past. There they acquire the authority of the time-honoured tale, the ancestral weight of everything that ever was. The very word 'once' is a story's equivalent to the knightly 'Sir' and the more elaborate 'Once upon a time' marks the newborn tale as a descendant of a noble house of story dating back to the beginning of time. You are knighting your new creation in the moment it is born.

To the story-maker, invocations are a personal mantra, a kind of alchemical formula for the successful distillation of tales, a catalyst for all that is to come.

It is good to have a store of such formulas at hand. You may like to begin all your stories with the same invocation, or you might want to experiment with different formulas for different tales.

Another strategy is the ritual of silence. Silence is indispensable in the spontaneous telling of story. A great gift to any writer, silence is the story medic's stethoscope, the instrument that keeps us in tune with our tales.

By silence I do not mean the mere absence of sound, but the presence of active attention, the intensive listening that opens into inner space. It is this listening that makes a story reveal its tale. Use it as much as you can and it will save you from any lack of plot. Give in to it and it will give you what you most need: the next step that your story wants to take, the turn your hero needs to make, the way your story longs to end. It will tell you everything and if it does not it may be that you have forgotten something on the way. The next chapter will help you to find it.

22. A Lesson in the Elements

Children live strongly in their imagination. Through imagination they add to reality what reality lacks. They see more than is there. Their imagination is playful and alive, just as they themselves are.

But childhood imagination does not just exhaust itself in mere fancy. It also serves as a means of perception for invisible companions, companions that only the child can see. To the child their presence is as real as that of a family pet. Children commune with their invisible friends through the language of childhood, that mixture of innocence and wonder that widens their awareness beyond the limitations of the adult world.

This same condition of soul allows children to encounter the world of elemental beings: the gnomes, dwarves, trolls, manikins, fairies, elves, tree men and well women, nixies and river-gods, wind spirits and thunder giants that populate the kingdom of childhood. They are more than mere fancy. They are the generic experience of children the world over. In the recent past their presence was a matter of fact in European folklore. To the medieval alchemist they were as tangible a reality as the substances of the elementary table are to the contemporary chemist. Most tribal societies are still acutely aware of these beings and relate to them through elaborate ritual. Elemental beings belong to nature long before nature became the abstraction we know nowadays. They are an essential part of the pre-intellectual world.

The World of Elemental Beings

Confronted with the abstract mind, elemental beings hide behind the formal contours of the world, the semblance of nature. Or they preserve themselves in folktale and myth and in the minds of those whose imagination has stayed most alive: the great poets. You can find them in Shakespeare's *A Midsummer Night's Dream* and *The Tempest*. In Goethe's *Faust* they appear in both their Nordic and Greek forms. They are a frequent subject of Blake's poetry and cause trouble in Ibsen's *Peer Gynt*. The fairytale derives its name from the presence of these beings.

To the child they are an undivided part of all-encompassing nature.

To the storyteller they are a great gift. Elemental beings greatly enlarge the repertoire of our tales with imaginal realities familiar to the child. If you invite them into your tales, they will most likely come. Elemental beings love stories — tales are one of their few remaining refuges, and often their only means to enter our adult life. They are always keen to join our heroes and help them on their way.

But they are not only of help to our heroes. They bring gifts for the storyteller too, and hide them in unexpected places: in the nooks of time and the crevices of soul. You may not find them immediately or even know they are there. But in your next tale, or the one after that, you may chance upon them. You may not know why your story took such an interesting turn, why the telling was so much easier than usual and why it all ended in such an extraordinary way. You may be puzzled as to where this story came from and surprised at your emerging gift for making tales.

No matter whether, or how much, you intend to invite fairies and gnomes into your tales, it is important, at least once, to acknowledge their presence in story reality. To ignore them is a major mistake. If as story-makers we do not call on them, we deprive ourselves of a crucial stage in imaginal development and all the help and direction it provides.

The Water of Life

The opening of the German folktale The Water of Life bring us an elemental lesson in imaginal conduct.

> There was once a king who had an illness, and no one believed that he would come out of it with his life. He had three sons who were much distressed about it, and went down into the palace garden and wept. There they met an old man who enquired as to the cause of their grief. They told him that their father was so ill that he would most certainly die, for nothing seemed to cure him. Then the old man said, 'I know of one more remedy, and that is the water of life. If he drinks of it he will become well again, but it is hard to find.' The eldest said, 'I will manage to find it.' And went to the sick king, and begged to be allowed to go forth in search of the water of life,

for that alone could save him. 'No,' said the king, 'the danger of it is too great. I would rather die.'

But he begged so long that the king consented. The prince thought in his heart, 'If I bring the water, then I shall be best beloved of my father, and shall inherit the kingdom.' So he set out, and when he had ridden forth a little distance, a dwarf stood there in the road who called to him and said, 'Whither away so fast?' 'Silly shrimp,' said the prince, very haughtily, 'it is nothing to do with you.' And rode on. But the little dwarf grew angry, and wished an evil wish. Soon after this the prince entered a ravine, and the further he rode the closer the mountains drew together, and at last the road became so narrow that he could not advance a step further. It was impossible either to turn his horse or to dismount from the saddle, and he was shut in there as if in prison. The sick king waited long for him, but he came not.

Then the second son said, 'Father, let me go forth to seek the water.' And he thought to himself, 'If my brother is dead, then the kingdom will fall to me.' At first the king would not allow him to go either, but at last he yielded, so the prince set out on the same road his brother had taken, and he too met the dwarf, who stopped him to ask whither he was going in such haste. 'Little shrimp,' said the prince, 'that is nothing to do with you.' And he rode on without giving him another look. But the dwarf bewitched him and he, like the other, rode into a ravine, and could neither go forwards nor backwards. So fare haughty people.

When the second son failed to return, the youngest begged to be allowed to go forth to fetch the water, and at last the king was obliged to let him go. When he met the dwarf and the latter asked him whither he was going in such haste, he stopped, and said, 'I am seeking the water of life, for my father is sick unto death.'

'Do you know, then, where that is to be found?'

'No,' said the prince.

'As you have borne yourself as is seemly, and not haughtily like your false brothers, I will tell you how you may obtain the water of life. It springs from a fountain in the courtyard of an enchanted castle, but you will not be able to make your way to it without this iron wand and two small loaves of bread I shall give you. Strike thrice with the wand on the iron door of the castle and it will spring open. Inside lie two lions with gaping jaws, but if you throw a loaf to each of them, they will be quieted. Then hasten to fetch some of the water of life before the clock strikes twelve else the door will shut again, and you will be imprisoned.'

The prince thanked him, took the wand and the bread, and set out on his way. When he arrived, everything was as the dwarf had said ...

Story-makers can easily find themselves caught in a tight ravine. Like their heroes they can get stuck in the middle of nowhere, in the dead end of their adventure. They can lose their plot and not find it again.

Like the two haughty brothers, such storytellers have probably missed something along their way. Eyes fixed on inheriting the kingdom of story, they do not heed the little man on the roadside. They do not deem him worthy of attention and so incur his wrath. Their tale has ended before it properly began.

It is the little dwarf on the road who points the youngest son into the direction of his adventure. It is he who instructs him with the plot for his story, the way in and out of the castle, and gives him the very tools with which his quest can be accomplished.

He will do the same for you if you care to stop, show him the respect he deserves and make him party to your plans. That is as much as to say: let him into your story.

Attracting Fairy Folk

Just like the Water of Life, a good story is not easily obtained. The hero in search of it needs all the help she can get. As you do. So stay for a while with this kind of story and invite all the elemental help it may provide.

For the best way to attract fairy folk is by means of invitation. And the best way of issuing such an invitation is to bring them to mind. And the best way to do that is through revisiting your own childhood, that freshest part of yourself, the youngest child in the kingdom of your soul — the one who will not ignore the helpful folk that are waiting along the way.

If you don't have memories of fairy folk, make them up. Most likely the memories are deeply buried, or your intellect has blotted them out. Use your imagination to recall what you may have forgotten. This preliminary exercise will help you to befriend these beings again and contact the layers of your soul to which they feel akin. Here is a story by Annie Wearne who remembered her encounter with one of these beings during her childhood in England:

> I went down the concrete path from the back door.
>   Just beside the dingle-dell I stopped.
>   I know exactly where I saw him. There, sitting on a big white rock, on the left side of the path, was a Gnome. He was just like in the pictures: A bright green jacket, scarlet cap, long brown pants and shiny black boots (or maybe they were brown).
>   He was sitting with one leg crossed, resting on his other knee; just sitting. And he had a long white beard, so he definitely was a Gnome!
>   He didn't say anything; he wasn't especially looking at me. He was just there, in the dingle-dell, among the plants, on the big white rock.
>   I ran to get my mother, but when we came back, he had gone.

> Now that you have made contact you can invite them into your tales. Let your hero have an encounter with these beings. You will find their help always forthcoming. Elves come in handy to mend stories as well as broken hearts and trucks as in this story by Kay Rosen:

Once upon a time there lived a boy called Alexander Edward Montgomery. He had a number of wooden trucks and trailers and engines and cars but his very favourite was a big red truck he called Move It. He played so often with Move It that one day the big black wheel came loose and rolled off and the wooden strut that held it in place just splintered and Move It crashed into the wall and cracked right through. Alexander Edward Montgomery was devastated. He cried and cried and cried and his mummy tried and tried and tried to comfort him.

But the more his mummy tried to tell him he could get another truck the more he cried because he wanted only Move It.

That night he took the shattered red truck, the black back wheel and the broken wooden pieces and put them at the end of his bed. In the morning there it was just the same. He left it there for a night and a morning and another night and a morning, seven times over.

On the seventh night when Alexander Edward Montgomery was fast asleep a little elf found his way into his room through the window that was slightly ajar to let in the night breeze. The elf had heard Alexander Edward Montgomery crying from far far away but it had taken him seven nights to work out just where Alexander Edward Montgomery lived.

'Ah,' he said when he saw Move It in pieces at the end of the bed, 'I have just the thing.'

He took out his special elf glue dust and glued Move It together perfectly and dusted it down and he slipped away in the night leaving only a little sticky jam footprint on the top of Move It. Elves like sticky jam you know.

In the morning when Alexander Edward Montgomery awoke he couldn't believe his eyes. Move It was whole again. 'Who did it? How could it be?' he called out excitedly. His mummy came running and was just as excited — and then they saw the footprint.

You may use traditional elemental beings or make up a new one. They all have their place. You may find that trolls appear more readily on the steep slopes of Norwegian fjords, that fairies have a preference for English fog and gnomes for outcrops of the Alps. Location matters, but even in Melbourne, Australia, leprechauns might leap to the sound of an Irish accent. In this case they are part of the internal geography, the inherited landscape you carry in your soul.

It is also good to find new names; the old names have a tendency to become clichéd. They may not match your surroundings. Nordic dwarves seem out of place in the Australian bush. Let the landscape you live in inspire you to an authentic response and find new names and forms for old themes. Listen for a name that may be appropriate. You might hear it whispered on the wind as Suzanne Smith did:

Amber woke up. She could still hear the drums and the singing. She thought it had just been a dream. But she could hear them calling. It was dark outside. Amber went to the window and looked out. She could see all the stars and a white moon like a hole in the sky, making a great light.

Amber moved quickly. She crept out of her room and climbed through the cat door. There was a soft breeze and it blew against her bare arms. She heard it rattle through the trees.

'Everything is alive,' thought Amber, and at that moment she heard giggling. She looked up in the night light, and saw children flying in the wind. It seemed that the darkness shone right through them.

Amber was astonished and rubbed her eyes to look again. When she opened her eyes two wind children were standing next to her on the verandah. They giggled and looked at her with big friendly eyes. 'Will you come and play with us,' they said. 'We are meeting at the dam because tonight we are making a dust storm.'

Amber was surprised. She saw a picture of a dust storm in her mind. One that whirls through the day time, picking up dust and swirling it about in the distance.

The wind children giggled again and beseeched Amber. 'Please won't you come. It will be such fun and we will be back by morning.'

Amber looked out at the night. She could see the long grass swaying in the breeze and hear the trees whispering. It seemed they were calling to her. She felt the wind warm and gentle on her face and saw other wind children flying through the air so happy and bright. She wanted to join them.

'Okay,' said Amber, 'I do want to go with you.' So the wind children took her by the hand and she raced across the night and up into the air. There was a lot to see but it went by so fast that Amber was happy when the wind children put her down on the side of the dam.

There she could see where the drumming noise was coming from. Kangaroos and wallabies were thumping their long feet on the ground in a rhythm. She looked at the banks of the dam and yabbies were gathered there clacking their pincers in time with the beat.

Everything was alive.

With the help of such elemental beings, the imagination does more than walk on water — it takes joyous flight.

Closely related but not always identical with elemental beings is another band of invisible friends and helpful allies — the inner storytellers.

Inner Storytellers

Inner storytellers bring powerful inspiration. I came upon these most helpful folk in Nancy Mellon's wonderful *Story Telling with Children.*

To find your inner storyteller, simply imagine a character you would like to hear stories from, perhaps the kind of storyteller you wished for as a child. We all carry such storytellers in our imagination: it may be an old Aboriginal woman sitting in front of a fire or a New York taxi driver; a pipe-smoking sailor spinning his yarn or a Chinese sage. You will find your imagination full of mavericks eager to tell their tale. They can be readily called upon and easily befriended.

The inner storyteller can also oil the rusty cogs of the imagination when people are just beginning in story medicine. You may like to invoke a new narrator for each new tale or return to a particular trusted voice in the imaginal realm. There are many ways to work with this crowd of tale makers.

The Irish are a nation of storytellers. Kathleen Shiels called upon her Irish ancestry in the next tale:

> Kate Hallinan tugged at her shawl as she stepped out onto da narrow cobbled lane. Da strains o' da fiddle from the public house next door played hide and seek with the wind as she strode toward Meg O'Shaunessy's window.
>
> Feathery rain blessed her face and lightness of step graced her feet. For sure 'an it's da night for Kate and Meg to while away da hours wid tales o' da little people, da cruel coastal cliffs an' da mysterious mounds an da bog.
>
> Ah how grand to sit by da fire trading tales deliciously wrapped in words secretly old and deep, boldly fresh and brand new …

Once you have called them to detailed attention they will be ready to tell
you a tale. Usually it is the one you need to hear. Fairy folk are a great
help in this respect. They love to tell stories that take us on a journey which
only they can bring our way. That is if you can find them. But you surely
will if you look long enough like Janet Blagg for her Green Man:

> Look for a trail of leaf litter, a little mud, a smoothed out hol-
> low where recently he took his rest. There is nobody to be seen
> at first glance, but you know he's there. You sit down, compose
> yourself, then look around you with wide eyes that can feel the
> breeze on them.
>
> And there he is — how did you ever miss him? The Green
> Man is sitting ankles crossed in front of him at the base of a
> large tree, as old as anyone's grandpa, eyes bright yet shad-
> owed, smiling cheeks deeply lined and faintly verdant. A
> carved stick leans beside him, two snakes encircling its handle.
> He twirls a green felt hat in his hands.
>
> There's only one thing to say and you say it. 'Tell me a
> story.'
>
> 'That's the way to begin,' he laughs, and as he does a leaf
> falls from his mouth and his green tongue flickers. You can see
> he is full of humour, but easily you can imagine him solemn
> too, grave with stories of tragic consequence and irredeemable
> sadness.
>
> 'I'll tell you a story about Efegenia Pye, a girl after my own
> heart,' he says. 'The sort of girl you could call on in the middle
> of the night and take on a magic carpet ride.'
>
> And here's the story, just the way the Green Man tells it:
>
> Somewhere, in a town not far from here, in a house in
> a street that's almost the same as yours, but not quite, the
> Princess Efegenia is sleeping. I am flying through the night
> on my magic carpet, over the ocean, over the dunes, now over
> the low hills sprinkled with houses. It's not far now, and I lean
> to one side to make the carpet circle over the town in spiral-
> ling swoops till I can see the big tree in the back yard, the red
> tin roof of the house. It's very quiet, very dark, except for the
> moonshine.
>
> I bring down the magic carpet in the long cool grass of the
> back yard and see the cat vanish over the fence with a terrified

backward glance. Don't worry, she'll be back, she likes to know what's new.

I creep up the garden path to the back door and reach for the handle; luckily it's not locked. C-r-e-a-k. Now up the stairs and third door down, it's open. I stand in the doorway. There is the bed, under the open window and the billowing curtains blowing in the breeze. And there is the princess, she's murmuring in her sleep, she must be dreaming.

I go up close and put my head down next to hers and whisper, 'Efegenia, wake up. Wake up Princess Effy. I've got a big surprise for you.' She rubs her eyes and opens them sleepily. 'Oh it's you,' she says, and a question mark creases her straight dark eyebrows.

'Shh. Come with me.'

And Princess Efegenia slips out of bed in her pink pyjamas and pads after me down the stairs and out the back door. I take her hand in the darkness till we reach the magic carpet nestled in the long grass. Her eyes grow wide and a smile stretches across her face. I sit down and pat the carpet next to me. 'Come on, let's go.'

She holds on to me tight as we take off, up, up, over the rooftop. She looks down and leans over to point at her bicycle leaning against the back steps, gleaming in the moonlight. The cat pops its head over the fence. Then we are flying over the hills, the dunes, the sea, with the wind in our face and our hair streaming out behind us.

23. The Alchemy of Metaphor

The Seed Metaphor

Imaginal allies and inner storytellers are seed metaphors. A seed metaphor is a picture that contains many others. Like any seed it can grow into a mighty tree bearing the fruits of many tales.

C.S. Lewis started his *Chronicles of Narnia* with such a seed metaphor: the picture of a faun holding an umbrella. Lewis carried this picture for years. He planted it in the fertile soil of his soul and watered it with his imagination. Eventually it sprouted into the story of *The Lion, the Witch and the Wardrobe,* then branched into the other six books that comprise the *Chronicles of Narnia.*

Your ally is your first acquaintance with a living, independent metaphor. She opens the door for you, into the realm of the imagination. The imagination is wholly metaphorical, composed of pictures rather than concepts, processes rather than products.

By definition, a metaphor is 'a figure of speech in which a term is applied to something to which it is not literally applicable, in order to suggest a resemblance.' If someone suffers a nervous breakdown and we call him a ruin we have used a metaphor. We could also call him a wreck. Both are metaphors, but pointing in different directions. Ruin implies a longer process in time, a slow falling apart. A wreck may be caused by a storm, an accident or a sudden change of fortune.

Both words invoke pictures and pictures are always complex. A ruin stands on solid ground, but it may be on top of a hill or deep in a valley; in the middle of a city or on a crumbling cliff. It mentally invokes a whole landscape. A ruin may be of bricks or stone. It may be bleak or overgrown with ivy and moss. It may be surrounded by a few trees or a dense forest, shrouded in mist or in an open field beneath a cloudless sky.

Every metaphor is like an unfinished painting that finds completion in the mind. It is not fixed like a concept. It remains open and freely associates with its kind. Every metaphor has its own aura of meaning. 'Ruin' has a very different circle of friends and relatives from 'wreck.' It will more readily attract some metaphors while it rejects others.

Every metaphor is a seed for itself and the soil for another. Metaphors sprout in each other's presence. Even a ruin comes to new life in the right company, and so do all concepts when they become metaphors. They break out of the solitary confinement of their literal meaning. They gain colour and life and start to breathe in the spaciousness of the imaginal world.

The Liberation of Concepts

I think it is clear by now that metaphors are not just artistic fancy or literary device. They precede concepts in the same way that imagination foreshadows reality and myths anticipate history. Concepts are dried up pictures, thoughts are confined imaginations.

Metaphors are our means to liberate concepts and resurrect some of the life they have lost. As soon as the bird of metaphor is freed from the cage of concept, it takes flight. Now an incident in our life, a conclusion we have come to or a situation we have grasped may reveal unexpected insights. We may be surprised by the kind of bird that emerges — a peacock blind to his own splendid fan, an eagle who has never soared the heights, a caged dove dying to be free. It might simply be a humble sparrow wanting to chat. Most likely, it will be a duckling seeing itself as a swan for the first time.

The ability to turn concepts into metaphor is the key that unlocks the cabinet of story medicine. It is the means by which an imaginal pharmacist prepares her healing balms.

The very process of making of metaphors — of translating thought into pictures — is in itself therapeutic, irrespective of what the pictures are. This translation does not always come easily to begin with, and may need some practice at the start. But we are not translating the original into a foreign language. We are merely returning an event to the language to which it belongs — restoring the poem from the prose it has become.

Making Metaphors

Metaphors are the vocabulary of the soul, the language of the imagination. If we want to travel with our heroes, we need to learn this language, or rather remember it again. It is the only tongue that is understood in all the provinces of story.

If metaphor is already your mother tongue you don't need my advice. But if you have lost this language you can relearn learn it in the stages set out here. To begin with, we acquire a craft. Eventually it will become an art.

First, find one or more metaphors for something concrete: a pen. Try to find an original picture that speaks to your soul.

> A sixth finger
> A writer's wand

Now a metaphor for something abstract: happiness.

> A new red bicycle
> A skipping child

And a metaphor for a more complex abstraction: a long sustained effort that led to no result.

> A returned manuscript
> Climbing the wrong mountain
> Navigating with a broken compass

Now play with metaphors for the open road, a piano, a chair; a happy day, a depressing week; a metaphor for love, for the self, the soul; for gladness, for hate; for yellow, red, blue.

Once you have mastered this level of translation you are ready to translate a soul-problem into the language of metaphor. Alejandra Czeschka has done that in a simple story that addresses the issue of envy in the friendship of girls:

> High in the sky two stars play happily every night … that was
> for a long time! Until one dark night, when both stars shone
> the best, another one came and wanted to join the game.
>   That pleased one of them very much. But the other one was
> afraid the new star would shine the most.

The story translates the problem into metaphor and so contributes to the healing. There is no need to find a solution, to console or to give good advice. It is enough for the hero to be confronted with her own story. Like the heroes discussed in the first part of the book she hears her tale told. She will be able to accept in the language of pictures what she would otherwise reject.

Using metaphor in this way we have already stepped over the threshold into the use of therapeutic tales. In the next chapter we will fully enter this domain.

24. The Healing of Harms

Preventative tales may be the most important of all healing stories. Told at the right time they address problems before they arise. Such stories are a form of immunization for the soul.

Many of the ancient myths were preventative tales in their time. Told at the right moment they still fulfil this function today. In Part Two, I showed how old tales can become preventative stories. Here we are developing the skills to create original preventative tales. Using the imagination in this way will help you to address issues before they occur. The preventative tale is a particularly good way for parents to support their children.

No other period of life is as labour intense as the early years. During this time every story is a catalyst of change, a midwife assisting in constant rebirths. Childhood is a series of revolutionary changes with the repeated breakthrough of mind over matter that accompanies the child's Herculean labour through each new phase, step, challenge and possibility. Stories prepare children for the tasks ahead. They give the soul the direction it needs to find a way through the labyrinth of life.

But stories are not only given in preparation for a challenge. They can also be applied in the midst of crisis or after the fact to address unresolved crises, incomplete changes or stagnated development. These are therapeutic stories.

The Therapeutic Story

Therapeutic stories are tailored for specific situations. Depending on the issue, more or less imagination may be required to assist the healing. Let us start where it is most simple: with the many small accidents that are part of a child's way into adulthood.

The best way to address an accident is to retell it, along with everything that happened in its wake.

> The piece of bread that wanted to be cut and eaten; the knife that was just there and how it slipped and cut and made Annie's fin-

ger bleed until she cried; how she had to be taken to the hospital down the road and how the nurse looked at it and disinfected the cut and covered it with cotton; how the nurse's name was Annie too and how she knew Annie's Auntie Lynn, who was a nurse at the same hospital before she went to live in Brisbane.

Each little narrative detail acts like a bandage around the accident and further closes the wounds of body and soul. *The way home via the pharmacy and the special meal that Mum made that night and the pudding that wobbled so much that everyone laughed* — these are the last healing touches on the way back to normal. This kind of story will help the child to revisit the trauma until it is quite digested.

The healing of small cuts, burns and bruises, of a broken leg or a twisted ankle, can be accelerated with a carefully applied balm of words. The many minor accidents that scar a child's life can be directly treated with the tincture of story medicine. They long to be acknowledged and celebrated. Every wound is an awakening. Boys and girls are often covered in bruises and are secretly proud of the calligraphy of scars scored in the playground. They are part of the body's rituals in its meeting with the world.

With more traumatic injury, the emphasis of story needs to shift towards the aftermath rather than the event and its causes; towards the healing that follows the accident. I suggest you bring in a hero to take the brunt of the event. The hero experiences a similar trauma to the child's affliction, but in metaphoric reality.

Jennifer Kornberger told the following story when her five-year-old daughter broke her lower jaw in a bicycle accident and had to have it wired to her upper jaw for six days:

> Once upon a time there was a man called Asep who had a beautiful lion. The lion ran freely in the fields and orchards and at night slept near his master's bed. Now one day Asep had to journey over the sea to the city where his brother lived. He packed his bag with bread and honey and healing oil. The lion asked to come with him, but Asep said that too many people would be afraid of the lion's jaws. The lion asked again, but Asep said the captain of the ship would not let a lion aboard. The lion asked a third time and Asep sat to ponder.

Finally he said, 'If you come with me on the ship you must
travel in a cage.' The lion who had never been in a cage said,
'Yes, I will come.'

When they came to the ship, the captain pointed to a cage
at the end of a deck. 'Put that lion in the cage there,' he called.
The lion went into a tiny cage and Asep placed six small
stones in the cage.

The waves heaved the ship up and down and water sprayed
over the cage. The lion could not stretch or walk and its head
drooped. But every day Asep came and sat next to the cage and
sang to the lion. And every day he took one stone out of the
cage and told the lion that when the cage was empty of stones
he would be able to walk free.

On the sixth day Asep took out the last stone as they sailed
into the new port. There was a welcome party and the cage
was opened on the jetty. The lion walked out and shook his
mane. Then it trotted beside Asep all the way to his brother's
home, carrying the bottle of healing oil around its neck.

A story like this is a phial of healing oil that will hang around the neck
of the patient long after the accident is forgotten. Children gain great
satisfaction from this kind of story. 'By accident,' they become the centre
of much attention as well as physical and emotional care that is crowned
by the story medicine.

The impact of a healing story is always multiplied with the use of
metaphor. Metaphor transforms a high fever into a furnace that forges
the hero's old sword into a brand new weapon. Or the fever becomes
a wall of fire through which the hero passes unharmed on the way to
the treasure. The story of a beaver busily damming a swelling stream
to save the land from flood can address an entrenched pattern like
bedwetting.

Above all, metaphor is an ideal means to comfort the soul in moments
of distress. Carole Longden has done this in her story of little starfish:

Once upon a time in a small bay where the water was clean
and blue and life was abundant, by a rock near the shore there
lived a little Starfish. Every evening Starfish climbed high
onto the rock. She loved to shine by the light of the stars and
the silver moon as waves lapped gently over her. And then, as

the first soft hues of pink appeared in the sky at dawn, Starfish returned to the water.

Along came the night of the full moon. Moon glowed white and round and smiled upon the earth. Starfish was very excited and climbed high onto the rock, when suddenly her leg caught on something sharp, leaving a deep wound.

Starfish tumbled down down down all the way to the bottom of the sea. She tried crawling along the ocean floor but her leg hurt greatly and so she stayed still and quiet for a long time. She felt sad and lonely and frightened.

Suddenly there appeared a frantic little turtle followed closely by a hungry fish. Starfish lifted one of her good legs and let Turtle hide there. The hungry fish looked confused and swam away. Little Turtle thanked Starfish and asked why she wasn't on a rock shining. Starfish told him of her plight and Turtle promised her she would not be disappointed, then swam away happily.

Before long a group of colourful fish darting to and fro swam playfully all about her. Their shiny scales flashed in the moonlit water, and Starfish felt a little better. Then Octopus came by, glowing in the moonlit water and stretching his many tentacles gracefully about. He stopped to give Starfish a gentle stroke on her injured leg before carrying on his journey.

Starfish smiled softly to herself. Then she saw something very large coming towards her. It was Whale! Whale swam right by Starfish, her long sleek body covered in barnacles and glistening blue in the moonlight.

Starfish was sure that Whale was the most beautiful creature she had ever known. Then to everyone's delight, Whale sang. She sang of all the joys of life and love, and Starfish knew deep in her heart that Whale was indeed precious. Starfish began to shine and continued to shine all night long.

And every evening from then on, Starfish climbed out of the water, high onto the rock, and shone brighter than ever — by the light of the twinkling stars and the silver-crested Moon, as the waves lapped gently over her.

Imaginal Healers

Another way to approach the therapeutic tale is to employ the doll as a nurse. Dolls are always keen to help and even minor accidents are of major concern to them. So it is with all the other imaginal friends too. The little sheep in the corner is sympathetic and the panther is incensed. The teddy bears will postpone their appointments to show support. The dog said he knew about it as soon as it happened and the cat insists she foresaw it the night before.

A small knife can cut deeply into a child's life and cause heated discussions around the kitchen sink. Only the fridge manages to stay cool while the pots ponder it deeply under their lids. The couch is too sleepy to care but there is much talk among the spoons about who is to blame. The drawer keeps its mouth shut but inside all the knives are on edge.

No one, of course, is more qualified to assist in accidents and the recovery of illness than elemental beings. No one knows better than fairies how to weave the gossamer of enchantment around an aching wound. Elves are good for any kind of healing, gnomes are the experts on broken bones and twisted ankles, and temperamental fire spirits are eager to burn up infection with the bonfire of their feverish heat.

An illness may also indicate the right moment to loosen the reins of the centaurs and let them come to your aid. They know every remedy under the sun, when to apply it and why. Centaurs have stories for each ailment and are always ready to come galloping all the way from antiquity right into your tale. And if you are very lucky, Chiron himself might appear on the doorsteps of your story. Let him in.

The Laughing Cure

Humour is a great liberator, especially in our capacity to laugh at ourselves rather than others. It requires us to not be overly identified with the temporal and the accidental.

Humour is the mark of the mature adult. Kids have lots of fun, but they rarely laugh about themselves. Like many adults, they can do so only indirectly and when prompted by outer means. Comedy or slapstick can provide us with the distance we have not yet achieved.

Comedy makes everyone laugh at themselves. It helps us come to terms, albeit implicitly, with the miser in us who cannot afford the expense of humour. The humorous story has such an effect on the child and is a wonderful healing tool. It takes some practice to get it right, but is worth the effort.

In the humorous story, unsavoury traits can be treated with great effect. The story deals with problems indirectly. The rascally hero of the story is never the child itself; it is always some other boy or girl. And in the story, the hero takes this unpleasant characteristic to the utmost extreme. There is no need to limit your imagination to the constraints of everyday reality. We can take a trait further and further until it bursts like a balloon blown up beyond its limits. Take a vice far enough and it will collapse and fall into the pit of its own creation.

Children love stories of rough justice. Like the djinns in *The Arabian Nights* they start to quiver with excitement when they hear them.

Like all human beings, children crave self-knowledge, but they need it in an appropriate form. They are not yet ready to deal with the pain that is often stirred up by self-knowledge. Humour is the only way to address it safely as it substitutes the pleasure of laughter for the sting of knowledge. It gently awakens the child's inner witness to watch over their outer affairs.

Here is such a story that softens the blow with humour, by Leah van Lieshout:

> Katie was real smart. She knew all her times tables by the time she was six and she could name all the rivers in the world by the age of seven. As she got bigger, so did her knowledge, so by the time she was ten, she was a walking encyclopaedia.
>
> Whenever anyone needed to know something, it was easy — just ask Katie. For instance, you might want to know what the time is right now in China. Well, if you find Katie, she'll tell you. 'It's ten o'clock in the morning,' she'll say.
>
> Eventually people stopped going to the library or reading books or looking up things on the internet — they just asked Katie.
>
> Katie would wake early and by seven o'clock there would be a queue of folks needing information that snaked its way around the block four times.
>
> At dinnertime there were only fifty people left and by midnight at last Katie could go to sleep.

In this story there is no preaching of morals, no clever arguments, no good advice. This story simply shows and exaggerates, and so produces a humorous effect. The situation says it all. (There is no need to argue with a demon. Let him do it himself. He is good at it!)

There are many ways to apply humour to story. One student wrote about a greedy little girl who ate all the fruit. When she gobbled a banana, a banana appeared on top of her head. Every strawberry, peach and apple she ate appeared on her head too. Soon she was walking about with a veritable tower of fruit that everyone but she could see.

The tale took hold of imaginative reality and pictured it in a form that would delight children as well as produce a healing effect. Here is a story by Jennifer Kornberger that uses humour to address the speediness of an eight-year-old child:

> Fernando Mazzo was the fastest boy in the town. At breakfast time he would finish his last spoonful of porridge just as his parents were eating their first. He ran all the way to school and was always the first person there. He ran thirty-one times around the oval until his teacher arrived.
>
> The writing he did in his book was so fast that the words spilled over the edge of the page. The teacher turned around and said, 'Fernando Mazzo, catch those words.' The words fell onto the floor and started running out of the door. Fernando Mazzo sped after them. The whole class stood at the door and watched Fernando Mazzo try to catch his words. But when the words reached the end of the verandah they leapt into the sunlight and floated off in all directions like dandelion puffs.
>
> The school maintenance man saw what was happening and gave Fernando a long-handled net from the swimming pool. Fernando ran, swooping the air with the net, but the words were already too high.
>
> One of the words got snagged in a Banksia tree. Fernando climbed the tree and edged along the branch. But just as he leaned on the last part of the branch, the word became unstuck and floated up to the clouds. Fernando Mazzo climbed down. The maintenance man said, 'You will have to wait until it rains, Fernando, until you can collect your lost words.'
>
> On rainy days Fernando now walks very slowly to school. So far he has found three words.

Contrasting Stories

Another way to apply humour to habits is to make two stories, contrasting the vice with its corresponding virtue — again, without moralistic preaching. Peter Tenni illustrates this in his two tales about Frankie:

Frankie and his Marbles (1)

There was once a boy named Frankie who was a good marble player. The more he played the better he became and the more he wanted to win. He had the biggest collection of marbles in the whole school. Huge tombolas, tiny pee wees, cat's eyes and hundreds of other marbles of all colours and sizes.

Every morning before school, every playtime, and every lunchtime, he would play marbles. He would bring his bag of hundreds of marbles to school with him, and take home dozens more each afternoon. As he won more and more marbles it became harder for him to find anyone to play with, until one day, no one in the whole school, not even the grade sevens, would play with him. Frankie continued to bring his marbles to school every day, but his classmates were no longer interested.

One day after school, as Frankie was struggling up the hill to his house with his enormous bag of marbles, he dropped the bag and his marbles rolled off the footpath and down the drain on the side of the road, and down the hill out of reach.

Frankie and his Marbles (2)

There was once a boy named Frankie who was a terrible marble player, and no matter how much he played, he never got any better at it. But Frankie liked to play marbles, even if he always lost, because it meant he could be with the other kids.

Every morning before school, and every playtime, and lunchtime, he would play marbles. There was never any problem finding kids to play with, it was always easy to win against Frankie. And every afternoon after school, and every Saturday morning, Frankie would load up his bike and deliver newspapers up and down the streets. With the money he earned, he bought more marbles.

One day after school, as Frankie was preparing for his delivery run, he heard a strange rattling sound from the drain on the side of the road. He looked into the drain and saw hundreds of marbles collected there. Huge tombolas, tiny pee wees, cat's eyes and hundreds of other marbles of all colours and sizes. Frankie was always able to go back to the drain for more marbles, as the supply seemed endless.

Frankie is still no better at marbles, and still loves playing with the other kids.

25. The Laboratory of the Imagination

Applied metaphors are a powerful means of healing, but not the most powerful one. They are still a crutch. They help us to get up and even to walk away from problems that have kept us constrained. But they do not make us skip and dance all the way home.

To fully join the dance we need to leave all crutches behind. Metaphors and stories gained by way of translation are still tied to their origin. They often remain encumbered by the circumstance of their conception. Stories do not need to address problems in order to be born.

Stories need no excuse to exist. They do not have to have a purpose. They can be a free creation, a child of love rather than a child of duty. It is then that they may unfold to their fullest potential. Unfettered by circumstance, they spread their wings and fly the firmament of endless possibility. Such stories have no other intent than to be told. In having no direct aim to heal they are the most healing. With no purpose attached they can serve the deeper purpose. It is in this way that our craft turns into the art of telling of new tales.

From Metaphor to Imagination

Story-making is an alchemical art practised in the laboratory of the soul. The tale transforms both hero and story-maker in the telling of it. It is a process of purification in which the base metal of the intellect is turned into the gold of the imagination.

Such a story is like a dove that brings us the message we most need to hear, our true story, a medicine gleaned not from the shallow pronouncements of symptoms, but from the deeper dimensions of origins. To reach this we need to court our imagination further. We began to learn its language in the chapter on metaphor. Now we need to adjust to its customs and way of being.

The Heroic Landscape

The imagination lives in slow time. To meet and court it we need to do the same. We need to take time and proceed slowly. Rather than taking immediate hold of a hero and hurling her into a plot, we first take the time to establish the surroundings in which she can safely be born. We can do this by visualizing a landscape. This slows down the process of our imagination and gives the soul time to adjust to whatever story wants to be told. Our intellect is fast, it prefers arrivals to journeys and likes answers rather than questions. It is quick to provide solutions before they are even called for and is prone to finish off processes before they are properly begun. Little wonder the intellect often misses the plot.

The imagination, on the other hand, takes its time. It moves at the speed of soul and stops to look at all the pictures it finds on the way. Landscapes likewise have time. Glaciers and deserts are the hour-glass of the ages. Mountains rise slowly and oceans are infinite. Even racy New York is not in a hurry to be described and a busy street takes a long time to be penned. A medieval village may wait hundreds of years to appear in your tale. Even a small back yard may occupy your imagination in a large way.

Landscapes are soul-scapes. They are part of our interior alphabet that helps us spell out our moods and map the lay of the lands within our soul. Every landscape is a province of us; a vast, complex metaphor of meaning that the soul understands long before the intellect has any inkling. This is why landscapes are the perfect entry points into the realm of the imagination.

No matter whether you are making a story with someone in mind, or you simply need an entry point for your tale, a landscape will lead the way, like an invocation on a large scale.

The landscape you create at the beginning of your tale may not be important to the tale itself, but it may be very important to getting it started. Use landscapes as a creative device, both to slow you down to the speed of your imagination and to anchor it in detail. A landscape will provide the right surroundings for the hero. Above all, it will give you creative time to gather momentum for the rest of your tale.

Any kind of landscape can serve as a soul-scape. A vast white frozen expanse with a little hump of an igloo on the horizon; a grey castle set against heather and wind; a solitary mountain peak; a village at harvest time in the foothills of the mountains or terraced rice fields emerging from morning mist. It could be the Gobi Desert, a city ghetto, a garden in the likeness of paradise or a back yard in Sydney; indoors or outdoors, in the past, present or future; realistic or fictional. Landscapes are soul-scapes and soul-scapes are everywhere.

If your story is for someone in particular, hold that person in your mind's eye, picturing them in as much detail as you can. Be aware of any feelings that arise. Then let everything go and wait for the picture of a landscape to emerge. Gaze at this landscape and describe it in detail.

If the story you intend to make is not linked to any particular person or purpose, start with the ritual of silence. Give yourself time, listen to your soul and wait for the landscape to arise. You will soon find yourself in the midst of one. Here is the beginning of a tale by Nandi Chinna:

> The grass is brittle and dry. Red river gums stand like tired
> sentinels along the creek bed. In the paddocks close to the road
> the prickly barbs of scotch thistles have spread like a thick pur-
> ple carpet from fence to fence. Here and there an abandoned
> farmhouse sits sadly under an old peppercorn tree, doors and
> windows gaping like ghost holes, portals to another time when
> children ran in and out and cooking smells drifted into the
> evening air.

Distillation of the Hero

Once the laboratory of your soul-scape is well established, begin to condense the hero from out of his environment. He is, in fact, already there; has announced himself in seas, lakes or plains. He is already in the landscape in one form or another, ready to take shape in time and space. He may not be alone. Most likely he will be at the beginning of his quest rather than in the middle of it. Distil your hero slowly from his surroundings, as in this story by Pen Brown:

> It is a flat land, grass land with mountains in the distance, and
> a wide shallow river that has cut its banks so they drop down
> straight. There are smells of water and stone and sage, the in-
> toxicating smell of hot earth and hay, things drying slow, sweet
> and sleepy in the sun.

But the wind is cold and it lifts the long black hair of the
man. There is a halo of feathers round his head and beads and
leather braids on his arms and he sits on a horse without a saddle with only a piece of rope looped round its neck instead of
a bridle.

On his bare chest is a strap that goes under his arm and over
his back and laced into the strap is an oiled leather container
full of arrows (which are also clothed in feathers). The horse
has a long tail that brushes the grass and in it are tied beads
like red bees and small twists of yellow thread and in its mane
is tied the black wing of a bird.

The man and the horse are very still.

They are listening … listening to a far, faraway sound …

Once the hero has arrived, the story might well take off by itself. If it
does not, add the catalyst of detail.

The Catalyst of Detail

One way of bringing in detail is to expand the hero into his family. The
constellation of family members often pre-determines the nature and
course of the quest. A father who has never returned from a journey may
send him on his way. Poverty may send him into the world. A dispute to
be settled may add to the trial; a prophecy waiting to be fulfilled, a debt
to be paid, a promise to be kept or a deed to be done, as in this story by
Jennifer Kornberger:

He is a shambling long-haired youth with a face that is ready
to smile and a voice that rides high when he is excited and
low when he is calm. His clothes are ill-fitting and he seems
to have packets and wads strapped to his body under his garments. When he passes through the forest part of it seems to
sweep along with him as though the trees wished to follow in
his wake. His glance always rests on the furthest place. Houses
and rooms do not hold him for long, he prefers to sleep outside. He plays a tin whistle gaily or sadly as the clouds decree.
His name is Yentz …

Yentz left home in autumn with his mother's blessing. 'Your

feet are the same size as your father's,' she told him. 'Here are
a pair of his shoes. See how they fit so well. Now go, my son,
and see if you can find him for there has been no news whether
he is dead or alive all these years.' Yentz kissed his mother and
bade her farewell and promised to find news if he could. He
strode out of the village in his father's shoes and took the road
through the orchards. There were red apples lying beside the
road and Yentz stooped to pick them up. He put them in a little
sack he had tied around his middle. Then he came to a cross-
road. 'Well shoes,' he said, 'which road do we travel?' And the
shoes started south and Yentz was mightily pleased at the way
they knew where to go …

Magical shoes, tokens, talismans and other gifts are helpful objects for
heroes to find along their way. Such special gifts might be a raven that
speaks, a goldfish in a flask or the calling of a dream. It may be a sword
handed down for seven generations, a spell to make rain, the gift of being
able to hear the grass grow, a needle that mends everything, a compass
that always points in the right direction, a snapshot from the future or a
feather from the tail of the Phoenix.

Nor need you restrict your tale to such time-honoured accoutrements.
Feel free, like Julie Dickinson in the next piece, to use contemporary
equivalents to the magical gifts of the past — all the technological gadg-
etry of a modern child's fantasies.

As Danny Detective got onto his silver scooter, he pulled his
cap lower over his eyes. He checked his bulky pockets for
magnifying glass, handcuffs, ropes, notebook and invisible
ink pen and straightened his bulletproof vest. He inspected his
boots with the hollow heels which carried his lifesaving radio-
active transmitter. He scrutinized his watch and hoped the mini
camera was in good working order. His silver scooter roared
into life and he took off in a cloud of smoke…

Magical objects are magnetic. They attract adventures. Each gift contains
the map of its own future and is an element of the challenge it will help to
overcome. So let the gifts lead your story to where the hero needs to go.
They will surprise both you both. Perhaps your story is not even about the
hero. It may be about the one who gave the gifts. You never know.

Forging the Hero

By now you have probably gathered enough momentum for your story
to proceed. If your story has acquired a life of its own, let it unfold. Let
the hero take you to wherever she fashioned her sword. Do not interfere
with her plans, but follow her footsteps and mark where they lead.

If your hero has not yet found her way you can point her in the direction of her quest. You may even lead her to the challenge that will change
her, at least for the first couple of tales. Heroes need practice. If a male
hero is lost, you could try a female one. They often know what to do.

Another useful device is to ask the hero for her story. She may have had
her adventure already and is just waiting for someone to share her tale.

If all the magical compasses, maps, signposts and bird-guides, companions, talking horses and flying carpets, VWs and tiger moths, newspapers from the future and mobile phones with a direct line to the muse
have failed to lead your hero into the thicket of adventure and back, try
feeding her on the archetypal fare of dark woods and castles, giants and
fairies and dwarves; lead her into the complications of a labyrinth or
let her parachute on to an unexplored island. Bring her to a walled city
without gates, a riddle that cannot be solved or a seemingly impossible
task. (Heroes are used to those.)

Let your hero retrieve whatever she lost from a dark tower at the top
of a winding staircase. Most likely she will find herself on the way.
Confront her with two dragons so she can find a new solution to their
age-old plight, or apprentice her to a witch who can teach her how to
spin the yarn of her tale. If your hero survives all this without taking off
in some peak experience or gaining additional depth, you may have to
premeditate the adventure. This should only be done for practice purposes and abandoned as soon as possible.

One way of premeditating a task is by announcing it by means of a
prophecy or a challenge that is clearly spelled out. Perhaps a lost Queen
seeks delivery from the loom of her endless weaving: a hero capable of
finding the thread she has lost. A dream may have told her that such a
hero needs just this prompting to find her at the end of her tale.

Or maybe a king seeks a champion to challenge three formidable foes
that cannot be overcome by either valour or strength. Your hero might
be just the person to unnerve the foes with her unerring talent for delay
and distaste for combat. There are many ways to win battles and turn a
story into a new direction.

Once your hero has acquired a taste for adventure, you can abandon all planning. She will find her own way. Simply begin with a soul-scape and let the hero emerge complete with her tale. When you have learned to walk at the speed of your soul, and move in and out of the pictures that present themselves, you can discard the soul-scape too.

From then on you may start your story at any point. You have learned your trade. Your apprenticeship is at an end. You are ready to leap any hurdle that a story may put in front of you. You have grown wings after all and can become airborne at any moment you choose.

Story-makers who have reached this stage cannot wait to air their tales, some of which have been gestating for a long time. Often these are not children's stories. They are the first explorations into the mainland of tales, into the dense interior of soul, the forest of forgotten places and buried hopes, the temple of future intents. The story may be a tale made for this moment, or for someone else, perhaps a friend who can't hear it yet. It may be the maker's own map of tomorrow or a partner's life in a nutshell. Or it may be the beginning of a tale that leads to another and another until a whole epic stands finished on the bookshelf. Here is the beginning of such an adventurous tale by Mags Webster:

It is a jungle shivering with wet glossy leaves, roots and vines entwined, the earth moist and pungent, the trees plunging great roots into the ground. The air quivers with the hum of insects, giant dragonflies patrol the heavy atmosphere, their bodies slick and petrol-blue. Above, the canopy sways with monkeys, flying foxes and birds which scissor through the air in flashes of coral and sapphire and emerald, and loop their raucous chatter around the trees. The jungle smell is lush and toxic with decay, a scent that sticks to the skin. There is a sense of expectation tracking you, like a panther on heat.

And it feels as though you have been walking for hours, until you are as wet as the leaves and sticky with mud, flecked with fragments of bark; your feet have become alien creatures, blindly pushing their way through the resistance. And you are barely upright, the jungle has pressed down on you, even the sounds of the birds and the monkey chatter cannot be as loud to you as your own laboured breath, the agonised beat of your heart. If you were to meet another along the way, what would they see? A quasi-human, tide-marked with filth, almost naked, hair tangled with twigs and spider webs.

Let me past, let me past — you scarcely know that the words come out, but this is where you need to be, and you knew it would take almost all the strength you have to get here. And it feels so close, you have lived and breathed this quest for so long that when you stop the searching it will feel like a wound, you will ache with the loss of it.

It is just as you were told it would be. There is a light filtering through the undergrowth, a pale bluish light that makes ghosts of the leaves, and the air freshens somewhat, as though some giant hand had lifted the lid of the rainforest. It becomes easier to breathe, to stand upright, and you feel as though you can reclaim your humanness from the tacky clutches of the jungle. What was it you had to remember? Don't enter by the main path, enter by the fallen stone. Keep your gaze on the ground. And, most important, pick up the feather before you pick up the key.

I can see the fallen stone, luminous in the strange light; and just beyond it, the dark yawn of the temple door. I must keep my gaze averted and make straight for the altar.

I step inside the door. All the jungle sounds cease, even the monkeys fall silent. The chamber fills with the eerie bluish light. There is the altar. And there upon it, a golden feather and a pewter key. I nearly have the key, I think, I just have to pick up the feather first. I stretch out my arm. The feather glows and trembles. But something is repelling my arm — as if my fingers carry a positive charge, and the feather likewise. My hand is attracted to the key as if to some powerful magnet, and only just in time do I stop my fingers making contact with it. I try again to pick up the feather, but the same thing happens. Hot tears spring to my eyes. I have toiled through the jungle, my brain burdened with warnings and counsel, I have been told again and again I am the chosen one, but nobody has told me I would face this challenge. Why? What have I been chosen for?

Perhaps to complete this story and follow it with others. For our stories need to be told. They are there for the world. We shall take up the tale for grown-ups in the final chapter, but first there is one last foray into the world of the child.

26. The Family Heirloom of Story

This chapter is devoted to a genre of stories that has almost become extinct — those in which parents share their past with their children. These stories are the most intimate form of learning. They wrap the child in a cloak of experience and provide a further initiation into the nature of time. Stories told by the mother and father are history lessons direct from the heart of those who experienced it.

The stories of our past stories map time for the child and make it aware of change. They provide the child with a greater perspective than the present can afford. They let the child inhabit another world and allow it to live a second life by means of the tale. It is also your chance to live the past again, creatively.

Your life stories are living memories infused with feeling, waiting to be told. They carry their own momentum. The sapling of your first story will grow into a tree, the tree into a forest and the forest into the landscape of the life you once lived.

Bring your memories to mind as clearly as possible. See them and feel them and your child will see and feel with you. Search for the details and bring them to life with elaborate descriptions.

There are two ways of telling these tales. The first is the Roundabout story.

The Roundabout Story

This kind of story is told around the child. This happens in any moment when the past becomes present, when the conversation turns toward what has gone before. An old story may arise at the dinner table; recollections are refreshed as memories are shared among friends or when the teapot inherited from Aunt Nelly brings to life the long-forgotten memory of afternoon tea and muffins on a starched tablecloth in Devon.

The past presents itself in many ways and wants to be shared. The more past we inherit, the more future we can expect. Once the sharing of the past was a matter of fact. Storytelling was a domestic art and so was conversation.

Sadly we are losing these arts to the monologue of the media. The voice of the past is obscured by amplifiers and conversation gives way to the babble of talkback radio. Old tales are crushed by the news and the events of our childhood are overshadowed by world events. We have lost our oral tradition and with it the life of our memories.

Story medicine can play an important role in resurrecting the oral tradition. For our children are best nourished by what is truly human, present and real; by what is really there at this moment, this time and place. There is so much to talk about, share, give and receive. The memories that are not shared are doubly lost. To avoid this loss they need to be told to the child by way of the parent's story.

The Parents' Story

The stories told by the parent are an important gift. They are not foreign to the child, they are part of the family treasury of tales that have already shaped the parent and through the parent the child. They are intimate friends long before they are known. Not to meet these tales leaves a gap in the time-body of the child. The past remains blurred and the present unexplained. The family genesis is hidden, the ancestral song unsung.

Do not keep this blessing from your children if they are willing to receive it. Of course you will have to choose the stories carefully, and time them well. Treat them as you would any experience in real life. Share those that are appropriate. Leave out those that are not.

The young child wants to partake of the best of you, love what you loved, and admire what you have admired. He wants to kindle his spirit on the highlights of your life; shape his soul on whatever shaped you. Your stories provide him with a second biography and imaginative experience.

If the child is young he will want to hear of your adventures in the animated world in which he still lives. Here is a story by John Hamersley in which he remembers the Gum Tree Man of his childhood:

> I had to be alone. The Gum Tree Man would never show up if others were present.
>
> The Gum Tree Man made it exciting to go by myself along the sandy bush tracks leading away from home. There was only bush, no houses and no people, but the tracks curved and

it was not possible to be sure what waited out of sight round
the next bend.

It was exciting, but could I become lost by going so far from
home along these unused lonely tracks? Somehow I knew the
Gum Tree Man would not let me get lost. He would wait round
the corner and when I needed him, he would be there, pointing
the way home.

Of course I did see the Gum Tree Man. He was covered in
gum leaves and did not look quite like other people, and he
was always high up in gum trees, not any other kind. He was
there, but I don't think everyone would have been able to see
him. He only allowed special people to see him.

I liked him a lot. He was a special friend.

Another way to start is to choose an incident from the time in your past
when you were as old as your child is now. Whatever interested you then
will most likely interest him now. Here is an example by Aidee Sherrie:

When I was as little as you, I had a big wardrobe full of dolls
all to myself. There were more than a hundred and I know
that because I used to count them often. A few of my special
dolls had names. In fact, they had seven or eight names each. I
kept sheets with their names written on them, adding to them
and changing them. My three favourite dolls were Teeny Tiny
Tears, Cathy and Nikita. I would spend hours playing with
my dolls. I would open the doors of the wardrobe and it was
big enough for me to sit in there. I would have tea parties with
them, wash and dress them and even sew new clothes for them.
Cathy's dress was particularly beautiful and I remember hand
stitching around every single flower printed on the material.
On Sundays I would have a little prayer service for my dolls. I
would light a candle and sing. When I grew up I decided that
it was time for me to pass on my dolls to my younger sisters.
And when my sisters grew up, they passed those dolls onto
their children and they are still looking after them today.

If you are a parent your stories are an important part of the ancestral tale.
Told as they are by the tale's very hero, they provide a double intimacy.
They are the most personal of tales. Such stories can be any length and

can be made from even the smallest fragments of memory, as in this story by Leanne Sutton:

> When I was a little girl and started school, my mother would pack my lunch with Vita Wheats. Each morning I would squeeze the vegemite and butter through the holes in the biscuit. Then I would sit down and count how many black worms came through and how many white worms came through. There were always more white worms and I licked them off last.

Stories like that are big events in little lives. Simple as they are, they contain a great deal of observation. They are part of the exploration of childhood. The next story, written by Tom Muller, is a perfect story for a father to pass on to his son.

> When I was little, I used to collect tadpoles from the garden pond and place them in a glass bowl in my room. I watched them grow over the weeks. And one day the tadpoles, who had developed little legs and lost their tails, started jumping out of the glass bowl into my room. They were everywhere. I caught as many as I could and released them back into the wild. The tiny frogs seemed happy and vanished into the woods.

Almost anything is story-worthy. The way you arranged your room as a child, your many adventures with your dog, the stamp collection that was the best in the neighbourhood, the tricks you played on Dad, the odd habits of Aunt Nancy, the sewing of dolls' clothes, the making of cubbies and airplanes, all the small and large adventures in the bush, and the journeys to and from school. We forget how rich our lives have been. The sharing of your own tales will help you to remember. The content of the stories is obviously important, but equally so is the act of telling, the time together, the communion with past.

One way to enter the labyrinth of the past is by means of a thread that leads you back to where you have come from. This thread may be found in the china that came from England when your grandparents left for Australia on a ship that nearly sank in a storm. The three perfectly shaped pebbles you found on the same beach you met your husband. The old cupboard that has been in the family for five generations, and the trusty fridge that followed you from Sydney to Perth. The complete works of Shakespeare bought in Stratford-upon-Avon, a kimono purchased in a back street in Tokyo and the eagle's feather you found in the Sierra Nevada on a trip with a friend. These are all threads of your life, your biography. A small box you treasure may contain not only the history of you, but other stories as well, as in this beautiful example from Leanne Sutton:

> When my Pop was alive he did not have a lot of money. He would cut all the buttons off his worn out shirts. He would collect buttons from wherever he could. When we walked to the shops he would use his eyes like a hawk to see if there were any on the sides of the road. If he found one he would put it in his pocket and later place it in a blue cardboard box in his laundry. Later, when Pop went to heaven, your uncle lived in that house but he never knew about that blue cardboard box. Then I lived in Pop's house and one day when I was cleaning the cupboard I found the blue box. I lifted the lid and inside were scores and scores of buttons. Gold and silver ones, flower and boats, round and square and so many different colours …
> And now my child, you may choose a button from pop's blue box to sew on your purse.

The thread here is simply a cardboard box. But with story, it is a treasure chest. A casket of family jewels could not be more precious. It is filled with imagination, a good part of the essence of grandfather's life, a history lesson and a teaching more valuable than a lot that we learn in school. The button the child chooses will be a special gift, a blessing that links her to the ancestral story that will continue to be told through her life.

Grand and Grander Tales

Standing on the pedestal of the past, the stature of grandparents surpasses ordinary size. Their lives are already surrounded by the aureole of 'Once upon a time.' Your parents may or may not have been heroes to you, but to their grandchildren they are semi-mythical figures, particularly if you know how to select the best of their lives for the stories you tell.

The storyteller's memory of his own mother will be precious to the child. To the child the grandmother is the matriarch of the family line and deserves to be acknowledged in tales. Pen Brown celebrates her mother in this tale:

> Mum reads.
> Mum reads out loud.
> Mum makes people and mountains leap off the page.
> I've lived in the desert and lit fires by rubbing sticks and watched a witch doctor point a bone, and I've slayed a dragon, been befriended by talking animals, I've discovered a magical pearl in the throat of a fish. I've climbed mountains to a glass palace and run from robbers with their daggers drawn and had a wish granted by a genie and flown in a plane. I've done all this in the safety of the big stuffed armchair, tucked under Mum's arm, helping her turn the pages.
> My mum bakes bread and cuts yellow cheese from the round in its muslin cover ...
> Everyone wants to come to my house to eat Mum's bread and the home-made jam and the yellow cheese cut from the round in its muslin cover ...
> My friends all want to be cuddled by my mum. They love her jokes and the way she lets us play in the creek and get all dirty without turning a hair, and the way she lets us splash our paints on the floor, eat all the fruit and build cubbies (dens) in the lounge room with all the sheets and pillows and the way she lets our cat have kittens. My friends can't believe it.
> 'We love your mum,' my friends say.
> 'Not as much as me,' I say.

The storyteller's father is an important cornerstone on which family story can be built. Tales about grandfather are soul-food for the child and worthy to be recorded in the family history of exceptional deeds. In the tale below Jennifer Kornberger describes her father Roy Cox:

> Dad had been conscripted into the army reserve as a young man. For two years he lived the army life: getting up early, following orders, saluting officers and sometimes playing pranks on his friends. Dad had a friend called Des who liked to sleep

in long after the siren. Dad grew tired of shaking him awake every morning so he came up with a plan to cure Des of his habit. One morning, Dad and few of his mates carefully lifted Des's bed, with Des fast asleep in it, onto the parade ground. Then they lined up for the morning parade, standing to each side of the bed, with very composed faces. Des woke up to the whole battalion standing to attention listening to the sergeant major.

When I was just your age, Dad liked to pretend to be that sergeant major. At bedtime he would call out, 'Stand by your beds,' in his best army voice. Except that Dad's voice always had a hint of a laugh in it. We would all run to our neatly made beds that Dad had built for us, standing tall, awaiting fresh orders. 'Prepare to jump into bed,' he called, and then, 'Jump into bed.' Next came, 'Prepare to go to sleep,' and 'Go to sleep.'

We shut our eyes tightly and giggled down to our toes as Dad turned off the light.

The great-grandparents have an even more wonderful ancestry. Their remoteness in time brings them even closer to story. A great-grand-mother that was already a semi-mythical figure from a golden age for the storyteller will be even more so for the child who listens to her tale. Here is such a story to lean on, by Adrian May:

When I was a little boy I used to wear flannel pyjamas in the winter time. I loved how warm they kept me, even when I was not in bed.

Some mornings when I would wake up, Nina, my grand-mother, would be playing the piano in the lounge room. If I put on my dressing gown and tied up the cord, she would put me on her knee and keep on playing. I loved to be between her arms and watch her fingers dance over the notes and the most beautiful music would well forth. I would close my eyes and lean back into her warm bosom and I thought I was in heaven!

The further back we travel in family, the more fabulous the stories become. Great-grandparents and even more ancient ancestors can open the floodgates of family imagination and myth. Already old when the storyteller was young, they are remembered from the perspective of a child. This makes them especially grand tales for children. Here is one such 'fabulous story' by Gaye O'Donnell:

> Great Grandma Halligan was a very tiny lady, under five foot tall she was, but her personality was so big that people thought she was over seven foot high, giant size. She was a complex woman, scary, beautiful, smart and strong. She was a Spanish lady with wild black eyes and matching hair, she was a stunner they said, a one-of-a-kind.
>
> She was so wise that people travelled for miles to see her and ask her advice, but they never stayed long, because she always seemed to know what you were going to say before you did, and you rarely got to finish a sentence with her around. She knew things she couldn't know and did things that she couldn't possibly do.
>
> Once, I saw her lift a car out of a bog without even getting her shoes dirty. My sister told me they flew to town in the wheelbarrow to get some sugar for her cup of tea and my dad says that when he was just a boy, Great Grandma would sing songs in Gaelic that put the household to sleep for days, just so she could get all her chores done in peace.
>
> She could boil a kettle by whistling and close the curtains with a blink. The beds were always made and not a dish ever lay in her sink.
>
> Sometimes, late at night, she would let me brush her hair, which was longer than she was, and she would tell me stories of the otherworld from which she came.

This is indeed a 'grand story.' Imagination and reality meet in marvellous magical realism that will delight any child or adult. You can take such tales as far back as your family history or your imagination will allow. A fabulous ancestry may be one of the ways to enter the imaginative tale.

Stories about Work

Few topics are as story-worthy as the work of the storyteller's mother or father. All work is sacred and every skill inspires awe.

Work is an expression of our ability to contribute to the world. Behind the mask of necessity lies a selfless act drawing on effort, skill and capacity. Early childhood is an age of matriarchy and the rituals of daily work are worthy to be counted among the heroic tales of motherhood. In the extended family, it might be the grandmother, as remembered by Meg Aldridge in this tale:

> Gran let me help her shuck (shell) the peas and eat the smallest one out of each pod. The shining green peas would bounce into the mixing bowl and as it became deeper I could put my hand in and feel their smooth skin against my fingers. When we had finished, and she had a cup of tea, I sat in the well of her skirt and her large arms cuddled me to her.
> 'My lovely helper,' Gran would say.

Stories about work prepare the child for life and stimulate the imagination with the possibilities the future holds. Children often admire adults for the work they do or the way they do it. Like Gaye O'Donnell, you will possibly remember someone you simply adored for the way they did their job:

> Gibby had always been old, for as long as I could remember.
> He taught me how to play pool before I could even see over the table. He showed me how to strike matches in a strong winter wind, he even told me how to roll a good cigarette — just in case I ever needed to know.
> He cut the hay at harvest time and told stories to the other old men at the bar of how I could run so fast through the paddocks that the snakes would never bite me. I loved him for all his character, but I never knew how much until that special day.
> There was a cow having trouble calving. It was her first calf, she was young and we were all worried. I had moved her into the cattle yards and Dad had called old Gibby to help. The calf was breech and that usually meant death for calf and sometimes mother too — rarely was there ever success.
> I watched Gibby carefully that day. Fag in mouth, talking so sweetly to that young cow as he pushed around her belly. He spoke softly as he twitched wire around the calf's hooves.

Telling her all the time what he was doing as though she'd understand. He hummed 'good girl' gently to her as he moved the calf around inside her. We all watched in awed silence.

I was his assistant, getting everything ready before he asked for it.

He twitched a large stick around the wire once the legs were in place, still whispering gently to the young heifer. He slowly and gently pulled that calf right out on top of himself, but it wasn't breathing.

'Hay seeds, mate,' he ordered, putting his hand out to me. I was ready. He pushed the seeds up into the calf's nose and squeezed its ribs with the other hand. It sneezed into life, violently snorting out the seeds.

Everyone laughed with relief, he patted the mother and thanked her and Dad patted his back and thanked him and it was beers all round, and much frivolity, but I never spoke, I stood there silently, quietly, next to a God.

From such tales, the path opens into a whole forest of stories. One memory will lead to the next, one incident invoke another. To a parent this offers a kind of biographical cure as the best parts of life are reassembled into a body of story. It is a chance to truly remember the best of oneself.

The Child's Story

The family history is complete with the youngest of tales, with stories about the child itself. Children (like most adults) love to hear stories about themselves. Some of their doings they may not even remember. Such stories are good-humoured and adventurous, and ideally begin with something like, 'When you were two years old ...' Jennifer Kornberger made such a story for her son Johannes:

When you were not one year old you crawled through every room in the house and opened every drawer that you could reach! You began in the kitchen. One by one you took the saucepans out and then the lids to the saucepans, until the drawer was empty. Then you started on the drawers with the tea towels and cloths. You crawled into the bedroom and opened the shoe drawer. You squealed with happiness when you saw the pile of shoes you had made on the floor and the clean, empty insides of the drawers.

In Waldorf kindergartens parents are often invited to join their child's birthday celebration and tell a little story from each year of their child's life. Such stories act like rungs on the ladder of time and secure the passage into the future.

Hearing one's own story being told is a deeply healing act. Remember how this was a catalyst in the lives of Odysseus and Parzival. Hearing one's own story is the core of story medicine. Through the child's story you can administer this medicine to your child and, through telling the stories of your own life, to yourself too.

27. Grown-up Tales

This final chapter focuses on stories for adults. Like King Sharya, adults need stories no less than children do. We live in a world of severe story deprivation and the effects are visible everywhere. The care of the soul has been neglected far too long. Individuals suffer as much from the lack of story as our civilization does.

Adult Tales

Most of the techniques described in the previous chapters can success-fully lead into adult tales. The following story by Janet Blagg is written for children, but with an eye for the adult reader to enjoy it too.

> Everything was quiet in the kitchen, all the people had gone to bed and turned out the lights. Suddenly there was a clatter and a crashing and the cutlery drawer burst open. The knife and the spoon were fighting again. All the cups and plates and dishes and pots sat back to watch and see who'd win.
>
> 'I'm by far the most important,' said Nigella Knife sharply. 'Without me to chop it up, nothing would even be small enough to fit in a spoon.'
>
> 'Oh that's very cutting,' said Lucy Spoon softly, 'but it's simply not so. Lots of things fit in spoons.' And she dipped herself into the honey jar and came out dripping a round glob of honey all over the knife.
>
> 'Now that's sweetened you up,' she said.
>
> 'Yum,' said the knife as she marched off to find some bread and butter to spread for a midnight snack, and everyone settled down again.

Imaginal allies and inner storytellers work equally as inspiration for adult tales. These characters can be as unconventional and eccentric as you like. Being a native to the imagination they can be drawn from the choicest traits that reality has to offer. The more detailed you see them the better for your story. Like the imaginal ally they thrive on attention and are willing to give what they receive. Here is a description of an inner storyteller by Mags Webster:

> Mr Harry Valentine is portly, dapper, short. Handkerchief in pocket. Has spent years trying to learn the clarinet. Drinks port and lemon — bit of a lady's drink — but it is what his mother always wanted, and Harry always took her to the Fox & Hounds each Friday for lunch. Lives alone in the family home now his mother has died, but keeps her ashes in a musical box on the card table in the corner of the lounge. He is 58 years old and has never had a lover, but has been in love many times. His favourite word is oleaginous, and his favourite author is Dickens. He gives up chocolate for Lent each year. He is addicted to crosswords. He is unable to sleep when there is a full moon.

Even the elemental world can reappear in new and unexpected ways in adult tales. If you have followed the steps outlined in this part of the book you will find it easy to attract them into your stories. Most likely they are already waiting for an invitation to come into your life. And they are always helpful, as this story by Meg Aldridge testifies:

> Lily White watched the footprints on the white sand fill and hold water in their well. Slowly the sea sank back into the moist grains. The tide came higher, rushing in, covering the footprints. Waves broke close to her, crashing on the beach, and she moved further towards the dunes to prevent the cotton skirt that almost reached her toes, from becoming wet. The breakers took hold of the dry seaweed and dragged it into the ocean and spat it back, wet and shining, onto the shore.
>
> Lily knew that if she was going out in the dinghy she should have pulled it onto the sand at low tide. By now she should be out beyond the waves — not allowing them time to control and rule her. Annoyed that she had hesitated, Lily hitched up her skirt and started to wade towards the boat.
>
> The cold water broke around her ankles. She took deep breaths and forced herself forward, felt the seaweed dragging on her legs. As she became deeper she turned her back towards

the waves as they broke. With regained balance she turned to
face them again and now with water above her hips she could
see the buoy and the dinghy tugging on its mooring line.

Looking out to sea, observing the dinghy in the distance,
she questioned why she had set herself such a worthless challenge. The thought took her concentration and a wave broke,
punched her squarely in the stomach and sent her toppling
and somersaulting under the surface. Lily could see the light
through the water and, with all the power she could muster,
forced herself up and gulped at the air but another wave, more
ferocious, followed, grabbed her and took her under. She
fought to the surface, struggling and coughing and cursing her
stupidity; confused and searching, desperate to find her bearing, she saw her.

Next to Lily swam a young woman — wetsuit clad — water
sparkling on her eyelashes — a face like Lily's, only youthful
— long limbs. Lily wanted to ask 'Who are you?' Lily wanted
to cry and be forever in the young arms that with a firm grip
pulled Lily beyond the waves and into the gentle swell of the
ocean. Together youth and woman held hands, floated, stared
up at the blue clear sky and giggled. Together they caught
a wave, lay flat on it, arms stretched forward with the spray
tingling their faces and rode it to the shore.

As Lily lay on the dry sand, content and grateful she turned
to thank the young woman but she was not there. But now Lily
knew where to find her.

And if you look long enough, you too will find the help you need to tell
your tale.

The sequence laid out in the laboratory of the imagination works just
as well for the making of adult stories. You can follow the same path
suggested there. Start with a landscape and you will soon find your hero
in it, as Dianne Marshall does in the beginning of her tale:

It is hot and dusty. The landscape is red, tinged with the blue
green of saltbush. The road too is red. It is dirt and rutted with
a sprouting of desultory plants in the middle hump. The shoul-
ders go up rather than fall away. It disappears in a straight line
towards the horizon. There are trees, but they're few and far

between and none by the side of the road. The only thing by
the side of the road is a woman looking hopefully under the
bonnet of the car, giving the impression that she'll know what
is wrong when she sees it. The truth is she won't. The truth
is she's hot and tired and frustration is creeping all over her.
She doesn't know what to do but thinks raising the bonnet will
illuminate her. At least she is doing something. The fact is she
has just been to town some sixty kilometres away to do her
weekly shopping; home is some sixty kilometres ahead and
she is stranded between the two ...

The background landscape of this tale not only helped to find the heroine
but also supplied the very predicament she is faced with. Once you have
arrived at this point the story will have enough momentum to proceed by
itself. If you need more inspiration add the catalyst of detail.

Janet Blagg began with the creation of a soul-scape then added first
the hero, then the catalyst of detail:

The Monastery Garden

Across the valley you can see the monastery spread out on an
acre of hillside. Alongside one tall building is a walled garden, its creamy limestone wall high and solid against the thin
blue sky. You enter through a solid gate. Within, a wondrous
juxtaposition of ordered form and joyous profusion of rampant
plant life. Old fruit trees in lines, a tangle of climbing rose that
is yearning for freedom and making its way over vegetable
frames to merge its fragrance with lavender and hollyhock.
Over by the kitchen door, the herbs, another wild profusion,
thyme gone mad with all sense of hours gone.

Overlooking the rows of tomatoes, their leaves pungent in
the sunshine, a wooden bench. On one side of it a sundial,
on the other a well. On the bench, head bowed, sits a young
novice, whose task is to tend the garden. His job is to reimpose
order that was let slip by the last gardener, an old monk who
let everything go to the glory of god.

With secateurs and pruning saw, Ivan is to remake the lines
of precision and curb and tame the rambling rose. He sighs.
There are roses in his own cheeks, an ardent foxfire in his

eyes. He loves the wildness and the heady mix of scents in the walled garden. He drops the secateurs and with long and sensitive fingers he feels for the locket at his throat, his mother's. It was her deathbed wish that he give his life to God. He opens the locket, where the faded portrait of her frail strength stares into the mirror image of his father's heavy brow. He lifts his eyes to meet the creamy perfection of the rose, rises and buries his face in its pale pink softness. Lifts his eyes again to the leaves of the tall trees moving in the wind beyond the protection of the high wall, fluttering and dancing in the breeze.

He kisses the rose, turns. His feet crunch on the gravel path, past the lozenge-shaped beds and ornamental pond, to the high gate. He takes the key from the chain at his waist, unlocks the gate, throws the key into the field beyond, pulls his cassock over his head and lets it drop to the ground, walks across the field diagonally, against the grain.

The making of therapeutic tales is important for adults and children alike. I have experimented with stories as healing modalities in adult life and have found that the artistic use of metaphor is the key factor in the therapeutic process. I have devised two ways to use metaphor as a healing tool. The first I call 'picture mining.'

Picture Mining

Picture mining is a freer variation of the healing metaphor. Here the picture need not relate directly to the situation at hand. It may be inspired by it, but it is not bound to it. Such pictures are best mined from the depth of the imagination rather than from the surface of symptoms. Ideally they are the response of one soul to another.

In picture mining you can apply all the skill you have learned in the laboratory of the imagination.

Begin with an inner picture of the person for whom the story is to be written. Be aware of any feelings that arise. Hold the feelings for a while and then let them pass. Empty your mind and wait for a picture to arise.

Here is one such picture mined by Jesse Williams:

In this land there stands a mountain, tall and strong, whose
roots go down deep into the earth, unshakeable. A soft breeze
blows, rustling the dry grass that grows upon the slopes. But
if you were to tunnel beneath this mountain, you would find a
massive cavern. The whole inside of the mountain is hollowed
out. There you would find a volcano by a lake, and beside the
lake a tall stone arch, with these words inscribed upon it: 'It is
unloving to want what another does not wish to give.'

Beneath the arch is a small boy, weeping.

Pictures, of course, need not literally be mined from the depths of earth.
They can be on the open sea, in a garden or a building. They can be a
description of a scene or they can be in the form of a story as in the following example by Desma Kearney:

The Little Wooden Boat and the Wide Wide Ocean

Once there was a wide wide ocean
that stretched its watery arms between one mountain and
   another.
The wide wide ocean was a thousand years across
and a thousand years deep.
Its floor was blacker than a starless sky
and colder than a sunless sea.
Its face was at times ferocious
and at times still as a mirror.
There floated on the wide wide ocean
a little wooden boat with a sail made of skin.
Its hull was old and smooth
and its bolts were rusted and salty.
The little wooden boat no longer remembered who had built
   her
who had sailed upon her
or who had cast nets from her prow.
As she travelled on the wide wide ocean,
carried by silent slipstreams and singing wind
the little wooden boat found out
which mountain kept the moon, and which the sun.
Through blue days

through nights full of eyes
through ink skies spreading like fingers
through the rumpus of waves
the little wooden boat sailed
the wide wide ocean.

Such pictures are maps traced from the recipient's own soul. They are soul-scapes that we can trust to show us the way to the heart of the hero. In picture mining it is best to let the imagination do its work, and refrain from trying to translate symptoms into metaphors. Simply tell the story and let it take care of itself. It will say enough and no more. The story may not even address the problem you had set out to address, but another you were ignorant of. It may start to heal a wound before it is even opened or complete a long process of healing you were not even aware of. And it may do none of that. It may simply be a means to be together, of addressing the wound of separation and healing it through the communion of the souls.

Communal Imagination

The communion of soul plays an important part in the making of healing tales. Most problems of the soul are processes in isolation. They have ceased to communicate.

Unlike the intellect the imagination is a master communicator. The imagination and the pictures it contains are sociable by nature and so set the precedent for the rest of the soul to follow. Good stories are particularly potent in this respect as they present a highly organized matrix of meaning in which all parts communicate. Meeting such stories helps the soul to orientate itself. The imagination held in such stories readily communicates itself to the isolated part of the psyche and so assists its re-integration into the whole.

Just as there is the potential of communion in imagination, so there is the potential to work with imagination in communion — or 'communal imagination.' In workshops it is often the case that unresolved issues resist transformation into metaphor. Problems often cannot be metamorphosed into story because we get stuck in the intellectual interpretations we impose upon them. It seems as though the interpretation is as much an issue as the presenting problem. Perhaps even more so.

This observation led me to experiment with communal imagination as a means to help dissolve the armour with which traumatic events surround themselves. By sharing painful issues with others and receiving their imaginal responses, thick walls can crumble and iron gates break open.

Receiving healing metaphor stories from others bypasses the fortress intellect and jumps the hurdles of rationalization. There is no need to dissolve with the intellect what the intellect has largely helped to create, to cure the soul with the poison that has caused its distress. All it takes is to speak to the soul in the language the soul understands, and bring imagination to bear on problems that have resisted solution in any other way.

In this process soul speaks to soul, and imagination to imagination. Imagination is naturally compassionate and possesses a wisdom of its own.

To harness this wisdom I have worked with small groups of between three and seven participants, each sharing a major life issue with the others and receiving their imaginative response in turn.

The process starts with all members setting down their issue in a paragraph or two in plain language. (Just this act of writing down should not be underestimated in the process of transformation.) Then one by one, each person then reads their issue out to the group.

The fellow writers now bring their imagination to bear on what they have heard. They follow their inner pictures and let them unfold. I encourage participants to take seriously whatever imagery their imagination presents them with and follow wherever it leads. The loops and turns the imagination may take are often surprising, sometimes strange and occasionally bewildering. But these seemingly strange turns often end up the most meaningful to the one for whom the story is made. In any case, the response stories produced by the group generally make immediate sense to the recipient, tailored as they are to her particular soul needs.

In the Metamorphosis process every participant is in turn the healer and the patient, and everyone is freed by the communion with others through imaginal means. There is a peculiar freedom, when writing for another, that bypasses the intellectual insistence on 'getting it right' that writers can experience when creating stories about their own issues.

This process of story-trading is obviously dependent on the ability to work with pictures and follow their lead. For anyone who has practised the path outlined in this book, or who is naturally gifted in the telling of tales, this is well within reach. In workshops with newcomers I first spend some time oiling the rusty cogs and gears of the imagination. It is often surprising how quickly imaginal capacity can be accessed.

My work with Metamorphosis is still in its infancy, and there may be a book dedicated to the process in the future. In the meantime, I am available to start groups on the process. For those who feel confident to begin immediately, partners may be found through our online campus for global creativity: *www.sofia.net.au.*

To fully appreciate the process of Metamorphosis, one needs to have personally experienced the give and take of stories in community with other. Here, though, are some examples of the work to whet the appetite of those who wish to pursue imaginal communion through story-making.

First, here is a summary of an issue shared by one participant during a Metamorphosis session:

> I fear I maintain a distance, disengagement, withdrawal from the world … a gate beyond which you may not pass. I don't know if it's existential aloneness or what keeps me mainly single. I'm not comfortable with raw emotionality or emotional demands and I worry there is something autistic in this; that my concerns are purely selfish. I do engage with others, for instance a refugee I see as marginalized in our society, and I think that without me there is no one for him here. But he is difficult and deep down I wish I didn't have to do it. But I don't have to; no one makes me. So maybe I project that ultimately there is no one for me, that when I die there will be no one to empty my cupboards or treasure my books and files and writings.

The two stories that follow are responses to the issue above. Naturally they are most meaningful to the writer who shared her issue. But we can nevertheless gain an inkling of their healing potential.

Driftwood by Harriet Sawyer

> Once upon a time when the sun was as insistent as a cicada, and the sand lay like a marble slab, and the sea was as green as malachite, a driftwood raft appeared on the horizon. No one knew where it came from but the villagers swam out and

pulled it to shore. On it, there was a salt encrusted child clasping on to a silver book. Her hair had grown green as the malachite sea and her fingernails shone like pearls. How beautiful she is thought the villagers, and though the fish were scarce the women fought amongst each other over who would take the beautiful child home. Finally it was decided that Zania, who had no children of her own, would be entrusted — the others sighed as they wished for a girl whose fingernails shone like pearls — but they realized that this was the best way, and went home to their fishnets and urchins.

The girl was named Driftwood after the raft that brought her. She soon became part of the village — mending the nets, scaling fish, and helping with the washing of the boats. Soon everyone forgot that she had not always been there. However, there was one thing that set Driftwood apart. She never, ever, uttered a word from the moment she arrived. She smiled and played with the other children, and she sang the songs that brought the rains down and the fishing boats in. But never, ever did she speak.

Zania grew to love the child as her own, and wondered why a girl so loving and bright had been rendered mute. The one day she found Driftwood huddled near a lamp in the corner of the room. She was trying to hide a squid she had pulled in and was milking for ink. Zania was curious. The next day, when Driftwood was cleaning the boats, she searched the room. Finally she found beneath the bed a pen and ink in a small earthen pot. And when she lifted the mattress there were at least ten books of the sort you could buy at the market, with thick parchment paper. Driftwood had filled nine of the ten books with curious scribbles and nearly filled the last.

The poor child, thought Zania, remembering that Driftwood had come from far away. But what to do? A child cannot be forced to speak.

Zania had an idea. She had kept the silver book that the child had been clutching when she arrived. Each night, while the nets were being mended, she opened the book as she told stories of her own girlhood, of the whale they found, of the orange robe she had worn on her twelfth birthday, and how she had thought that her mother was the moon's sister. One hundred, two hundred, three hundred stories she told. And when no story, no matter how small, was left, she sat by the fire and she too ceased to speak.

Driftwood gathered up her books, and at the market she gathered as many beautiful glass bottles as she could find. Each page she ripped from the books. She folded and rolled and sealed each in a bottle with cork and wax. One hundred, two hundred, three hundred bottles she finds and fills.

She launched the fleet on a day when the sun was as insistent as a cicada, the sand a marble slab, and the sea shone like malachite. And when she returned home, she smiled at the old whitewashed door and said, Good morning mother.

The Train and verse by Deb Mickle

The train is at the platform. There is moderate activity, neither hectic nor frenetic. The sun is warm and the air has brightness. The train will depart soon, people get on and take up their seats.

This train has compartments, there is a separateness possible. Some people find this familiar and comfortable.

But there is an open carriage too, all the seats without walls, everyone's bags, cases, pillows, all visible. Less private, less sheltered.

She sits in a closed compartment and readies herself for the journey, prepares for non-engagement, the automatic part of her. Other people come in to the compartment. A few are in the wrong seat and leave. The train leaves the station.

She has planned to use this time to write, to be comfortable and purposeful. The writing is interrupted by a question from a passenger across the compartment. Surprise and annoyance. The question is answered — it rattles the writing mood. The train stops and people leave and get on. The compartment consists now of only her and the person who asked the question. Liberty to talk more? What choice will she make?

> There is moss and dew
> all fresh and untouched
> viridian green moss with no sign of day on it yet

all dewy and glistening
a jewel of preciousness
we walk around this moss and this place
with gentleness
knowing this is fragile, bringing no harm
and we leave it untouched
the moss and the dew
to repeat its cycle
reclusive and self sustained

We live in the middle of a story that demands our collaboration. To tell this story we need to continue the tradition of spontaneous storytelling and parable making. The making of stories is not restricted to poets and writers. The imagination is waiting to awaken. Its fruits can be reaped if the right steps are taken. To encourage the taking of these steps was the aim of this book.

Bibliography

The Power of Story

Barfield, Owen, *Poetic Diction: A Study in Meaning,* Wesleyan University Press, Middletown, 1973.

—, *Romanticism Comes of Age*, Wesleyan University Press, Middletown, 1986.

—, *A Barfield Reader*, ed. G. B. Tennyson, Floris Books, Edinburgh, 1998.

—, *History in English Words*, Lindisfarne Press, Hudson, 1967

—, *Saving the Appearances: A Study in Idolatry*, Harbinger, New York.

—, *Speakers Meaning,* Wesleyan University Press, Middletown, 1984.

Barks, Coleman (Trans.), *The Essential Rumi*, Penguin Books, London, 1995.

Bullfinch Mythology, Modern Library Paperback Edition, New York, 1998.

Fridell, Egon, *Kulturgeschichte Griechenlands*, Verlag C.H. Beck, Munchen, 1976.

Gilgamesh, see Sandars

Graves, Robert, *The Greek Myths*, Penguin Books, 1992.

Homer, *see* Riev

Houston, Jean, *The Search for the Beloved*, J. P. Putnam Sons, New York, 1987.

Larousse World Mythology, Hamlyn Publishing Group, London, 1973.

The Odyssey, see Riev

Ovid, *Metamorphoses*, Viking Press, New York, 1958.

Plato, *see* Tredennick,

Riev, E.V., (Trans.), Homer, *The Odyssey*, Penguin, London, 1991.

Rumi, *see* Barks

Sandars, N.P., (Trans.), *The Epic of Gilgamesh*, , Penguin Classics, 1960.

Shakespeare, William, *The Complete Works*, Magpie Books, London, 1992.

Sophocles, *King Oedipus*, Penguin Books, Harmondsworth, 1947.

—, *Antigone*, Penguin Books, Harmondsworth, 1947.

Steiner, Rudolf, *Theosophy: An Introduction to the Spiritual Processes in Human Life and in the Cosmos*, Anthroposophic Press, Hudson, 1994.

—, *The Kingdom of Childhood*, Anthroposophic Press, Hudson, 1964.

Tarrant, Harold, *see* Tredennick

Tredennick, Hugh, and Tarrant, Harold. (Trans.), Plato, *The Last Days of Socrates* (Apology), Penguin Books, London, 1993.

Uehli, Ernst, *Mythos und Kunst der Griechen*, Philosophisch–Anthroposophiser
    Verlag, Dornach, n.d.

de Waal, Esther, (Ed.), *The Celtic Vision: Selections from the Carmina Gadelica,*
    Darton, Longman and Todd, London, 1987.

Zaehner, R.C. (Trans.), *Hindu Scriptures*, Dent, London, 1968.

The Making of Tales

Baldwin Dancy, Rahima see Dancy

Burkhard, Gudrun, *Taking Charge: Your Life Patterns and their Meaning*, Hawthorn
    Press.

Carlgren, Frans, *Education towards Freedom*, Floris Books, 2008.

Chilton Pearce, Joseph, *see* Pearce

Crowley, Richard, *see* Mills

Dancy, Rahima Baldwin, *You Are Your Child's First Teacher*, Celestial Arts,
    Berkeley, 1989.

Estes, Clarissa Pinkola, *Women Who Run With the Wolves*, Rider, London, 1992.

de Haes, Daniel Udo, *The Young Child*, Floris Books, Edinburgh, 1986.

Howard, A.C., *The Recovery of Man in Childhood*, Myrin Book, New York, 1989.

Koch, Kenneth, *Wishes, Lies and Dreams*, Harper & Row, New York, 1970.

Koenig, Karl, The *First Three Years of the Child*, Floris Books, Spring Valley, 1969.

Lievegoed, Bernard, *Phases of Childhood*, Floris Books, Edinburgh, 1987.

—, *Phases*, Rudolf Steiner Press, London, 1979.

—, *Man on the Threshold*, Hawthorn Press, Stroud, 1996.

Mellon, Nancy, *Storytelling with Children*, Hawthorn Press, Lansdowne, 2000.

—, *The Art of Story Telling*, Element, Melbourne, 1998.

Mills, Joyce C. and Crowley, Richard J., *Therapeutic Metaphors for Children*,
    Brunner/Mazel, New York, 1944.

Moore, Thomas, *Care of the Soul*, Harper Perennial, New York, 1992.

O'Neil, George and O'Neil, Gisela, *The Human Life*, Mercury Press, Spring Valley,
    1990.

Pearsall, Paul, *The Heart's Code*, Bantam Books, Milsons Point, 1999.

Pearce, Joseph Chilton, *Magical Child*, Plume Books, London, 1992.

—, *Evolution's End*, Harper, San Francisco, 1993.

Peck, M. Scott, *The Road Less Travelled*, Arrow Books, London, 1983.

—, *The Different Drum*, Simon and Schuster, New York, 1998.

Richards, M.C., *Toward Wholeness*, Wesleyan University Press, Middletown, 1980.

Sawyer, Ruth, *The Way of the Story Teller,* Viking, New York, 1962.

Strauss, Michaela, *Understanding Children's Drawings*, Rudolf Steiner Press, London, 1978.

Tacey, David J., *Edge of the Sacred*, Harper Collins, Sydney, 1995.

Winn, Marie, *The Plug-In Drug: Television, Children and Family*, New York, 1985.

Children's Literature

The Brothers Grimm, *The Complete Grimm's Fairy Tales*, Routledge and Kegan Paul, London, 1975.

Corrin, S. and S. (Eds.), *Stories for Five-Year-Olds*, Puffin Books, 1973.

Dante Alighieri, *see* Sayers

Ende, Michael, *The Neverending Story*, Penguin, London, 1984.

—, *Momo*, Puffin Books, 1985.

von Eschenbach, Wolfram, *Parzival*, Penguin Classics, London, 1990.

Graham, Kenneth, *Wind in the Willows* Simon and Schuster, 1981.

Green, Roger Lancelyn, *Myths of the Norsemen*, Puffin Books, London, 1970.

Grimm, *see* The Brothers Grimm

Guin, Ursula Le, *see* Le Guin

Jaques, Faith, *The Orchard Book of Nursery Rhymes*, Orchard Books, London, 1990.

L'Engle, Madeleine, *A Wrinkle in Time*, Bantam Books, New York, 1973.

Le Guin, Ursula K., *A Wizard of Earth Sea*, Penguin Books, London, 1973.

Lewis, C.S., *The Magician's Nephew*, Harper Collins, London 1992.

—, *The Lion the Witch and the Wardrobe*, Harper Collins, London 1992.

—, *The Horse and His Boy*, Harper Collins, London 1992.

—, *Prince Caspian*, Harper Collins, London 1992.

—, *The Silver Chair*, Harper Collins, London 1992.

—, *The Last Battle*, Harper Collins, London 1992.

Mackenzie, Donald A., *Teutonic Myths and Legends*, Gresham Publishing Company, London.

Matterson, E. (Compiler), *This Little Puffin, Finger Plays and Nursery Games*, Puffin Books, 1987.

Milne, A.A., *Winnie the Pooh*, Penguin Books, New York, 1992.

Pullman, Phillip, *His Dark Materials trilogy*, Scholastic, 1995–2001.

Russian Fairy Tales, Senate, London, 1995.

Sayers, D.L. (Trans.), Dante Alighieri, *The Divine Comedy*, Penguin, London, 1955.

Tolkien, J.R.R., *The Lord of the Rings*, Harper Collins, London, 1993.

Yolen, Jane, (Ed.), *Favourite Folktales from around the World*, Pantheon, New York, 1986.